Antibodies for Treating Can~

Melvyn Little

Antibodies for Treating Cancer

Basics, Development, and Applications

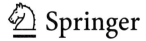 Springer

Melvyn Little
Sankt Peter-Ording
Schleswig-Holstein
Germany

Based on the German language edition:
Antikörper in der Krebsbekämpfung by Melvyn Little
Copyright © Springer-Verlag Berlin Heidelberg 2015. All Rights Reserved.

ISBN 978-3-030-72601-0   ISBN 978-3-030-72599-0   (eBook)
https://doi.org/10.1007/978-3-030-72599-0

This Springer imprint is published by the registered company Springer Nature Switzerland AG
The registered company address is: Gewerbestrasse 11, 6330 Cham, Switzerland

Dedicated to the memory of the late Jim Huston, creator of the single-chain antibody and founding President of the Antibody Society.

Preface

Nothing was known about the existence of antibodies when the first safe and effective vaccine against smallpox was tested by Edward Jenner on his gardener's son in 1796. It was only recently, about 200 years later, with a better understanding of the immune system and the biology of tumor cell development, that the first vaccines were developed against certain types of cancer.

The advent of recombinant DNA technology in the 1970s and the groundbreaking production of monoclonal antibodies by Köhler and Milstein in 1975 opened up an exciting era for developing antibodies to treat cancer. Their sequences were humanized to make them less immunogenic and functional features were optimized for mediating tumor cell killing. Emulating Paul Ehrlich's concept of "magic bullets," they were also armed with toxins and radioactive nuclides. To harness cytotoxic immune cells, dual-binding (bispecific) antibodies were created by joining domains directed against cytotoxic T lymphocytes or natural killer (NK) cells with antibody domains binding to specific markers on the tumor cell surface. In another approach, antibody binding domains were used to construct chimeric antigen receptors (CARs) for engineering cytotoxic T cells to target and destroy cancer cells.

Solid tumors are complex tissues often containing many different cell types that form the tumor stroma. An understanding of their interactions is essential for devising novel immunotherapeutic approaches. The discovery that the inhibition of the cytotoxic activity of tumor-infiltrating lymphocytes by the immunosuppressive tumor microenvironment could be blocked by antibodies against immune checkpoints (ICs) led to a breakthrough in the treatment of some solid tumors. A significant number of complete remissions have been achieved for previously recalcitrant cancers such as malignant melanomas and even lung cancers can now be treated with anti-ICs as part of a first-line therapy.

The goal of this book is to provide medical and biology students, lecturers, physicians, clinicians, and research workers with a concise description of antibodies being developed and used for the treatment of cancer. To demonstrate their potential benefits and possible side effects, I have summarized the results of clinical trials for a variety of approved antibodies. A short history of immunization and the elucidation of antibody structure and diversity provide a background perspective, and a short overview of the immune system facilitates a better understanding of antibody functions and novel immunotherapeutic approaches. I have also included several anecdotes to "humanize" various aspects of antibody developments.

Sankt Peter-Ording, Germany   Melvyn Little
January 2021

Contents

About the Author

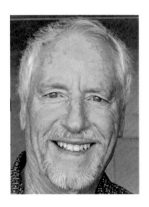

Melvyn Little

- B.Sc. in Chemistry and Ph.D. in Biochemistry, University College of North Wales, Bangor, UK
- Postdoc Max-Planck-Institute of Cell Biology, Wilhelmshaven, Germany
- Research scientist at the German Cancer Research Center (DKFZ) in Heidelberg, Germany
- Habilitation in the Faculty of Biology at the University of Heidelberg: "Structure and Function of Microtubules"
- External Professor of Biochemistry at the University of Heidelberg
- Head of the research group "Recombinant Antibodies" at the German Cancer Research Center, Heidelberg
- Founder and Chief Scientific Officer of the biotech company Affimed—Development of bispecific antibodies for treating cancer
- Currently retired and biotechnology consultant

Life-Saving Antibodies: History of Immunization

1

Abstract

In 1796, Edward Jenner scraped pus from the blisters of a milkmaid infected with cowpox, which he inoculated into the arms of his gardener's son to protect him from smallpox. Almost a century later, Louis Pasteur developed vaccinations against diseases such as anthrax and rabies using weakened pathogens. Shortly afterwards, Emil von Behring, Kitasato Shibasaburō, and Paul Ehrlich demonstrated that antitoxins in the serum of horses vaccinated with diphtheria toxin could cure diphtheria patients. The complementary lock and key binding of the antitoxin (antibody) with the toxin (antigen) postulated by Paul Ehrlich was confirmed 40 years later by Linus Pauling. As a direct result of the work of these early pioneers, successful vaccination campaigns have been carried out against various pathogens in the past 50 years. More recently, advances in the isolation and genetic engineering of antibodies against tumor-associated antigens have opened up new possibilities for treating cancer.

1.1 Introduction

One of the greatest achievements of modern medicine was the complete eradication of smallpox through a worldwide vaccination program. Can similar successes in combating cancer with vaccines be expected? Would it be possible to use the antibodies generated by vaccines for cancer therapy as in the original treatment of diphtheria? For better understanding the possibilities of vaccination and the recent innovative approaches in using antibodies to fight cancer, an overview of the historical development of immunization provides an interesting background perspective.

1.2   Variolation

Methods of variolation to immunize against smallpox (variola), which usually comprised inserting preparations of smallpox scabs or the content of pustules into small scratches, were practiced as early as the fifteenth century in China and somewhat later in the Middle East and Africa. The first medical account in Europe was published in 1714 by Dr. Emmanuel Timoni, an Italian living in Constantinople. It caught the attention of Lady Mary Wortley Montagu, the wife of the British ambassador to the Ottoman Empire, who was able to witness the process of variolation in Constantinople at first hand. She asked the Embassy surgeon Charles Maitland to inoculate her 5-year-old son Edward, so that he would not suffer the same fate as her brother who died from smallpox in 1713. She had also contracted the disease in 1715, which left her facially scarred.

Introduction of Variolation to England and Europe

On returning to England in 1721, Lady Montagu arranged for her 4-year-old daughter to be inoculated by Maitland. She then invited Sir Hans Sloane, the King's physician, to witness the result. His report aroused the interest of the royal family, particularly that of Caroline, Princess of Wales, who was acquainted with Lady Montagu. Charles Maitland was then granted royal permission to test the treatment on six condemned prisoners at Newgate Prison, who were offered a reprieve if they agreed to be inoculated. They all survived, and later one of them appeared to be immune to smallpox after being exposed to two infected children. The following year after the successful inoculation of Caroline's daughters, Amelia and Caroline, variolation became a popular medical treatment in England. Although some people still died after variolation, the number of deaths was significantly reduced by optimizing the technique, for example, by using only light scratches to introduce the inoculate of mildly affected donors. Impressed by the expertise of English variolators, Catherine the Great engaged the English physician Thomas Dimsdale to inoculate herself and her son Paul in 1768. The Russian nobility rushed to emulate their Empress, and Dimsdale, helped by his son, went on to successfully inoculate 140 people in St. Petersburg and 50 people in Moscow. Already a wealthy man, Dimsdale was rewarded with considerable amounts of money from Catherine and the Russian aristocracy and was granted a hereditary baronetcy with a pension for life. In the event that the inoculations would not be successful, Catherine had arranged for a relay of horses to take the Dimsdales out of the country.

Introduction of Variolation to North America

In the American Colonies, the New England Puritan minister Cotton Mather had read the publication of Emmanuel Timoni on variolation and learned the method from Onesimus, his West African slave. In 1721, during an outbreak of smallpox in

Boston, he tried to convince the medical community in Boston to inoculate the population. Only one physician, Zabdiel Boylston, agreed to test the new method. He inoculated his 6-year-old son Thomas and two Negro slaves. Boston's citizens were enraged, and Boylston had to go into hiding for 2 weeks. In the following spring, after the storm of indignation had subsided, Boylston defied an order of Boston's selectmen and inoculated 244 people. Only 6 died (2.4%), whereas 844 of the 5980 Bostonians who caught smallpox succumbed to the disease (14%). The procedure then spread rapidly to the other colonies.

Variolation of the Continental Army

In 1775, George Washington's Continental Army besieged British-occupied Boston, which was experiencing another epidemic of smallpox. Washington was very worried that his troops would get infected and he suspected that the British might deliberately try to infect his troops with the refugees that were released from the city. Around the same time, the Colonials advanced on Eastern Canada and managed to capture Montreal and began a siege of the fortress city of Quebec. If it had fallen, the British would almost certainly have lost Canada. However, weakened by smallpox, the Colonials had to retreat when the British reinforcements arrived. Washington, worried that his own army could be similarly decimated by the disease, finally persuaded the Medical Director of the Continental Army to inoculate his troops in 1777.

1.3 Vaccination Against Smallpox

A major advance in the fight against smallpox was the relatively harmless vaccination with pus from people infected with cowpox. To commemorate the first scientific vaccination with cowpox viruses in 1796, Edward Jenner donated the hide of the cow "Blossom" to St. George's Medical School in Tooting (UK), where he was a student and where it now hangs on a wall of the library. Blossom's fame resulted from the infection of the milkmaid Sarah Nelms with her cowpox. Edward Jenner scratched the pus from the blisters on Sarah's hand and inoculated it into both arms of James Phipps, his gardener's 8-year-old son (Fig. 1.1). Jenner later infected James on two separate occasions with smallpox, but no infection developed. He then systematically and successfully applied this procedure, which he called vaccination (vacca = lat. cow), to a large number of other people. Although Dr. John Fewster had reported 20 years previously on the ability of cowpox to prevent smallpox infection, an observation that was confirmed by several others in Germany and England, it was Edward Jenner's merit to clearly demonstrate immunity to smallpox by vaccination with cowpox.

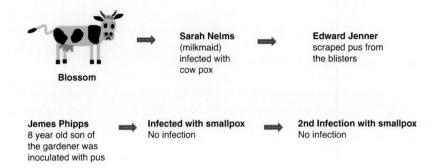

Fig. 1.1 Vaccination against smallpox by Edward Jenner in 1796

Eradication of Smallpox

In a unique worldwide campaign launched by the World Health Organization (WHO) in 1967, smallpox was completely eradicated. The last recorded case was an infected Somali in 1977, and in 1980 the WHO announced that this dreaded scourge of humanity had finally been defeated. The only remaining smallpox virus samples are kept for research purposes in two laboratories (CDC Atlanta in the United States and Vector Novosibirsk in Russia).

1.4   Vaccinations Against Other Infectious Diseases

Edward Jenner could only speculate on the mechanism of his vaccine. Nothing was known about the infectious agent. In 1864 Louis Pasteur formulated his germ theory, and in 1876 Robert Koch showed that bacteria were the cause of Anthrax (*Bacillus anthracis*). Four years later, Robert Koch provided evidence that tuberculosis was also caused by a bacterial infection (*Mycobacterium tuberculosis*). These findings were the final proof of the existence of bacterial pathogens. At about the same time in 1880, Louis Pasteur and his colleague Emile Roux showed that weakened chicken cholera bacteria could protect against virulent cholera bacteria. Pasteur managed to develop further vaccines against anthrax, swine erysipelas, and rabies. It became increasingly clear through his work that many infections could be prevented by vaccination. After successfully vaccinating the 9-year-old Joseph Meister against rabies in 1885, a wave of enthusiasm for his work culminated in a financial campaign to build the Pasteur Institute in Paris in 1887, which is still the leading biomedical institute in France.

The Tuberculin Scandal

As there were no rules at that time for drug trials, Louis Pasteur and Robert Koch were able to carry out clinical studies on patients, which were sometimes only based on assumptions and insufficient preliminary experiments. A particularly striking example is the tuberculin scandal in the last decade of the nineteenth century. Without convincing preclinical data, Robert Koch propagated vaccination against tuberculosis with a tuberculosis extract, which he called tuberculin. He also persuaded his 17-year-old lover Hedwig Freiberg to be vaccinated, pointing out that although she might get sick she was unlikely to die. There were some initial reports of successful vaccinations, but after an increasing number of deaths, its use was discontinued.

1.5   Healing Diphtheria with Horse Serum

Emil von Behring (a former student of Robert Koch), Kitasato Shibasaburō, and Paul Ehrlich were more cautious in testing their diphtheria antitoxin before administering it to patients in 1893. A series of detailed preliminary tests were carried out, and the results were extensively discussed with their colleagues. The aim of these experiments was not to induce an immunity to infection but to prevent the destructive effects of the toxin. Diphtheria patients were injected with the serum of horses that had been vaccinated with diphtheria toxin (Fig. 1.2). The serum neutralized the action of the toxin, and many patients were cured. A similar procedure was developed for the production of an antitoxin against tetanus. This was the first time that a so-called passive immunization had been demonstrated to save lives, for which Emil von Behring received the first Nobel Prize in Physiology or Medicine in 1901. Kitasato, whose part of the work appeared to be of equal importance, went empty-handed. He and von Behring coined the terms antibody and humoral immunity for the antitoxins produced in the serum. The protection by the antibodies usually only lasted a few months until the foreign proteins disappeared from the blood. Repeated applications are not possible because an overreaction of the immune system against the foreign proteins can lead to an anaphylactic shock with circulatory collapse.

With the prize money from the Nobel Prize, von Behring built the Behringwerke in Marburg, Germany, a pharmaceutical factory with a stable of horses for the large-scale production of serum.

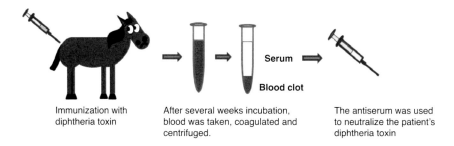

| Immunization with diphtheria toxin | After several weeks incubation, blood was taken, coagulated and centrifuged. | The antiserum was used to neutralize the patient's diphtheria toxin |

Fig. 1.2   Production of an antiserum against diphtheria toxin. A collaboration between Emil von Behring, Kitasato Shibasaburō, and Paul Ehrlich

1.6   Antigen (*Antibody-Gen*erating Substance)

To explain the formation of antitoxins, Paul Ehrlich developed a so-called side chain theory in 1897. He postulated that the toxins are bound by structurally complementary receptors ("side chains") on the surface of cells, similar to a lock and key. Since the receptors are important for the function of the cell, the cell tries to overcome the blocking effect of the toxins by producing more side chains. Excess receptors are then secreted into the serum as soluble side chains ("antibodies").

A first insight into the nature of antibodies was provided by experiments using an antiserum against pneumococcal pneumonia. Before penicillin was introduced, an antiserum was the only cure for this often fatal disease. In 1923, Michael Heidelberg and his mentor Oswald Avery showed that the antiserum bound to polysaccharides on the pneumococcus. Heidelberger was the first to apply mathematics to the binding of antibodies and antigens (the "precipitin reaction"), and he succeeded in precipitating the antibody with the polysaccharide antigen. After analyzing the precipitate, it was clearly demonstrated for the first time that antibodies were proteins. Michael Heidelberger continued to make important contributions to this field of research for an extraordinarily length of time. He was still working in the laboratory until shortly before he died at the age of 103.

The lock and key hypothesis as an explanation for the binding of an antibody with an antigen was confirmed by Linus Pauling around 1943. He found that the interactions depended more on complementary structures than on chemical compositions. The two binding sites of an antibody are identical and specific for a particular antigen.

1.7   Antibodies Are Produced in B Lymphocytes (B Cells)

Contrary to the earlier speculations of Ehrlich that all cells would have antigen receptors, he later assumed that only specialized cells in the blood plasma would produce antibodies. Almost half a century later, in 1948, Astrid Fagraeus showed in her doctoral thesis that plasma cells, later shown to be the matured form of white B lymphocytes, specialize in the production and secretion of antibodies. They are called B lymphocytes or simply B cells because they were originally first described in the *Bursa fabricii* (*Bursa cloacalis*), a lymphatic organ on the roof of the cloaca in birds.

1.8   Current Vaccines

The great strides made in immunization with non-infectious virus material over the past 50 years have led to the successful control of various diseases. Besides smallpox, the spread of the devastating infectious diseases polio and tuberculosis have been largely curbed by vaccination campaigns. Effective vaccines have also been developed against diphtheria, tetanus, pertussis (whooping cough), measles,

Haemophilus influenzae disease, meningococcal disease, and invasive pneumococcal disease to name just a few. A complete list of available vaccines can be obtained from the World Health Organization (WHO) and US Centers for Disease Control and Prevention (CDC) websites (see Selected Literature).

Effective vaccines have not yet been developed against the AIDS virus, the hepatitis C virus, and the malaria pathogen, in spite of enormous investments by national governments and philanthropists and intensive scientific research. In this global age, the emergence of other life-threatening viruses capable of rapid transmission across the world will probably happen at regular intervals. Mutations of relatively harmless viruses into dangerous pathogens are often made possible by the close contact between humans and animals. For example, in 1967, there was an outbreak of a new type of dangerous virus disease in the laboratories of the pharmaceutical firm Behringwerke in Marburg, Germany, which was founded by Emil von Behring for the development and production of vaccines or antitoxins. The virus, which came to be known as the Marburg virus, was found to have originated from imported African green monkeys used for animal experiments.

COVID-19 Vaccine

The corona family of RNA viruses also frequently causes epidemics of respiratory tract infections, some of which resemble the common cold and others showing more severe symptoms. Three potentially lethal members of this family have caused major outbreaks in the past 20 years: SARS-Cov-1 (severe acute respiratory syndrome coronavirus 1), MERS (Middle East respiratory syndrome), and now SARS-CoV-2 (severe acute respiratory syndrome coronavirus 2) causing coronavirus disease 2019 (COVID-19). The mortality rate of SARS-Cov-1 was estimated to be about 10% and that of MERS as high as 35%. Only about 2% of patients infected with COVID-19 die from this disease (depending on the quality of treatment), but it is much easier to transmit than the other two viruses, particularly in this age of globalization. While SARS-Cov-1 appears to have spontaneously disappeared and MERS seems to be under control, at the time of writing, the COVID-19 virus shows no signs of abating. However, in contrast to SARS-Cov-1 and MERS, the first effective vaccines based on mRNA coding for part of the COVID-19 virus spike protein have been developed by the firms BioNTech (Germany) and Moderna (USA) and approved within the record time of 1 year, an unprecedented achievement.

The virus was first discovered in Wuhan, Hubei province, China in late December 2019. A rapid response team was promptly dispatched by the Chinese Center for Disease Control and Prevention (China CDC) to accompany Hubei provincial and Wuhan city health authorities in carrying out an epidemiologic and etiologic investigation. RNA extracted from the bronchoalveolar-lavage fluid and culture supernatants was used as a template to clone and sequence the genome, which was made publicly available in January 2020. Using the sequence information coding for the spike protein, two vaccines based on mRNA in lipid nanoparticles (LNPs) developed by BioNTech/Pfizer and Moderna received Emergency Use Authorization

(EUA) from the Food and Drug Administration (FDA) and conditional marketing authorization by the European Commission within a year of starting development. Vaccines based on adenoviral vectors carrying DNA coding for the spike protein were developed almost as quickly (e.g. the vaccines of Oxford-AstraZenica, Johnson and Johnson, and the Russian vaccine Sputnik developed by the Gamaleya Research Institute of Epidemiology and Microbiology). More traditional vaccines based on the inactivated virus have been developed in China (e.g. CoronaVac by the Beijing biotech firm Sinovac) and a protein-based nanoparticle vaccine using the full-length, prefusion spike protein was developed by the US firm Novavax.

Ebola Vaccine

Close contact or consumption of wild animals also appears to be responsible for the transmission to humans of the devastating diseases AIDS and Ebola. In a recent Ebola epidemic, for example, the first outbreak of the disease was traced back to a 2-year-old child in Meliandou, a village in the hinterland of Guinea. A striking feature of this village is the frequent consumption of fruit bats, which are easy to catch in the adjacent trees. Some species of fruit bats are considered to be breeding grounds for the Ebola virus. Bats are also thought to be reservoirs for the coronavirus infections described above. In 2017, Chinese scientists traced the origin of SARS-Cov-1 to horseshoe bats in Yunnan.

Ebola, also known as Ebola virus disease (EVD), is a viral hemorrhagic fever of humans and other primates caused by ebolaviruses. The virus was first identified after the occurrence of an outbreak in Nzara (a town in South Sudan) and in Yambuku (Democratic Republic of the Congo), which is a village near the Ebola River from which the disease takes its name. It is a particularly lethal disease killing about 50% of infected patients. The latest outbreak, the 11th so far, occurred in June 2020 in Mbandaka, Équateur Province, a region adjacent to the Congo River. An Ebola vaccine named Ervebo was recently developed by genetically modifying the vesicular stomatitis virus to express an Ebola surface glycoprotein. It was approved for medical use in the European Union in November 2019 and in the United States in December 2019. It is not yet known how effective it will be in preventing disease.

Passive Immunization

The use of antibodies to neutralize infectious diseases has become increasingly important. Successful antibody preparations to combat Ebola, for example, have been generated from the B lymphocytes of an Ebola survivor and by the immunization of transgenic mice that produce human antibodies (see Chap. 5). More than 45 antibodies are currently being developed for neutralizing the SARS-CoV-2 virus. In November 2020, the FDA granted emergency use authorization (EUA) for both bamlanivimab (LY-CoV555) from Eli Lilly and the combination of casirivimab and imdevimab (REGN-COV2) from Regeneron in outpatients with mild to moderate

COVID-19 who are at high risk for severe COVID-19. REGN-COV2 became well-known a month before its EUA after being highly praised by President Trump who received a single dose of 8 g for "compassionate use" to treat his SARS-CoV-2 virus infection. The Regeneron antibodies were obtained from transgenic mice that had been immunized with the virus spike protein. They were selected for their ability to prevent the virus binding to an extracellular domain of angiotensin-converting enzyme 2 (ACE2), which mediates the entry of the virus into the cell. The data supporting the EUA for patients at high risk for disease progression showed that hospitalizations and emergency room visits occurred in 3% of the patients treated with REGN-COV2 compared to 9% for placebo-treated patients.

The development of vaccines to prevent and treat cancer is described in Chap. 3.

Selected Literature

Adler R. Medical firsts. 1st ed. Hoboken: Wiley; 2004.

Bishop WJ. Thomas Dimsdale and the inoculation of Catherine the Great of Russia. Ann Hist Med New Ser. 1932;4:321–38.

Boylston A. The origins of inoculation. J R Soc Med. 2012;105(7):309–13.

Coniff R. Stopping pandemics. National Geographic. Washington, DC: National Geographic Partners; 2020.

Corti D, Misasi J, Mulangu S, et al. Protective monotherapy against lethal Ebola virus infection by a potently neutralizing antibody. Science. 2016;351(6279):1339–42. https://doi.org/10.1126/science.aad5224.

Ehrlich P. Science History Institute. https://www.sciencehistory.org/historical-profile/paul-ehrlich.

Grundy I. Lady Mary Wortley Montagu. Oxford Dictionary of National Biography. Oxford: Oxford University Press; 2004. https://doi.org/10.1093/ref:odnb/19029.

Hansen J, Baum A, Pascal KE, et al. Studies in humanized mice and convalescent humans yield a SARS-CoV-2 antibody cocktail. Science. 2020;369(6506):1010–4. https://doi.org/10.1126/science.abd0827.

Henderson D. Smallpox: the death of a disease. 1st ed. New York: Prometheus Books; 2009.

Hopkins DR. The greatest killer: smallpox in history. 2nd ed. Chicago: University of Chicago Press; 2002.

Le TK, Paris C, Khan KS, et al. Nucleic acid-based technologies targeting coronaviruses. Trends Biochem Sci. 2021;46(5):351–365. S0968–0004(20)30295–4. https://doi.org/10.1016/j.tibs.2020.11.010.

Li Y-D, Chi W-Y, Su J-H, et al. Coronavirus vaccine development: from SARS and MERS to COVID-19. J Biomed Sci. 2020;27:104. https://doi.org/10.1186/s12929-020-00695-2.

Mortaz E, Tabarsi P, Varahramet M, et al. The immune response and immunopathology of COVID-19. Front Immunol. 2020;11:2037. https://doi.org/10.3389/fimmu.2020.02037.

Saphire EO. A vaccine against Ebola virus. Cell. 2020;181(1):6. https://doi.org/10.1016/j.cell.2020.03.011.

Silverstein A. The historical origins of modern immunology. In: Immunology. The makings of a modern science. 1st ed. London: Harcourt Brace & Company; 1995. p. 5–20.

US Centers for Disease Control and Prevention (CDC). https://www.cdc.gov/vaccines/vpd/vaccines-list.html.

Van Epps HL. Michael Heidelberger and the demystification of antibodies. J Exp Med. 2006;203(1):5. https://doi.org/10.1084/jem.2031fta.

World Health Organization (WHO). Immunization, vaccines and biologicals. https://www.who.int/teams/immunization-vaccines-and-biologicals/diseases.

Antibodies and the Immune System

2

Abstract

A basic knowledge of the immune system is essential for understanding the mechanism of therapeutic antibodies, particularly for the new generation of antibodies that are not directed against tumor markers but against immune checkpoints. This chapter illustrates the development of antibodies as part of the immune response and the interactions between components of the innate immune system such as monocytes and natural killer (NK) cells and components of the adaptive immune system comprising B and T lymphocytes. The major role played by cytokines in cellular signaling and regulatory mechanisms to prevent an overshooting immune reaction are also described.

2.1   Introduction

Antibodies belong to the so-called adaptive (or acquired) immune system. After vaccination with antigens from pathogens, it takes about a week for the production of antibodies able to fight the infection. Until then, cells of the innate immune system such as granulocytes, monocytes, and natural killer cells (NK cells) and soluble factors in the blood (the complement system) must keep the infection at bay. Macrophages (phagocytes) and the related star-shaped dendritic cells interact with the adaptive immune system by presenting T cells with phagocytized and processed antigenic material.

2.2   The Immune Response

The immune response is a fascinating series of finely coordinated events leading to the eradication of an invasive organism. For many years it was thought that the major trigger of an immune reaction was the detection of nonself material. A more convincing explanation was provided by the "danger signal" theory of Polly Matzinger in 1994, who postulated that the recognition of surface motifs on pathogens or alarm signals from injured or stressed cells by the innate immune system is a necessary requirement for an immune response. For example, after a bacterial or viral infection, receptors on macrophages and Langerhans cells (functionally immature dendritic cells within tissues) usually recognize a common molecular motif on the pathogen's surface. Binding to one of these receptors, of which there appear to be more than a hundred, triggers a series of signals that result in the differentiation of Langerhans cells to dendritic cells. After phagocytizing the foreign organisms and migrating to the T-cell region of the lymph glands, both macrophages and dendritic cells can present antigens from the digested foreign organisms to naïve T lymphocytes. Those lymphocytes with specific antigen receptors matching the peptide-MHC complexes (see below) on the dendritic cell are activated and differentiate to effector T cells, which then migrate to the site of invasion and attack the pathogen. Some of the T cells in the lymph gland differentiate to helper T cells, which can activate other immune cells, such as the B lymphocytes. Activated macrophages at the site of invasion send out signals to the endothelial cells lining the blood vessels which respond by producing adhesion molecules on their surface that facilitate the binding and migration of the highly mobile neutrophils through the tissue to the source of the invasion, where they aid the macrophages in fighting the virus. Later, they are joined by the activated effector T lymphocytes that migrate through the tissue by the same process. Finally, the activated B cells mature and differentiate to plasma cells producing high-affinity antibodies, which usually prove decisive in the final eradication of the foreign organism. Inhibitory feedback mechanisms prevent potentially damaging overreactions and ensure that the immune reaction is terminated after achieving its purpose. A more detailed description of the components of the immune system and their role in an immune reaction are given below.

2.3   Cellular Components of the Immune System

An overview of the cellular components of the immune system, which all originate from stem cells in bone marrow, is shown in Fig. 2.1.

Granulocytes, monocytes, and NK cells belong to the innate immune system. The most numerous granulocytes are the neutrophils representing 55–70% of the leukocytes (white blood cells). After recognition of the danger signals on the cell surface, the neutrophils ingest the pathogens by phagocytosis. After digesting the pathogens, the short-lived neutrophils die, and their remnants become the main part

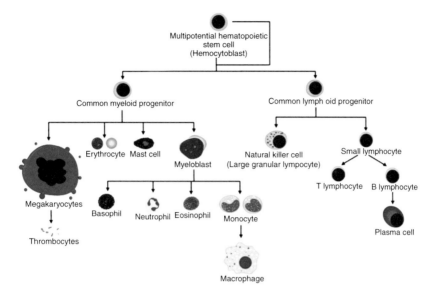

Fig. 2.1 Simplified hematopoiesis showing cellular components of the immune system. By Rad A and Häggström M. CC-BY-SA 3.0 license. https://commons.wikimedia.org/wiki/File:Hematopoiesis_(human)_diagram.png

of the pus. The rarest granulocytes are the basophils, which make up less than 1% of the leukocytes. Like mast cells, which reside predominantly in tissues, they bind IgE antibodies and play a major role in inflammation and allergic reactions. Both cell types contain granules filled with heparin and histamine. The eosinophilic granulocytes, which make up about 2–5% of the leukocytes, have a dampening effect on acute allergic reactions. They also contain a protein that is toxic to parasitic larvae (MBP—"major basic protein"). A more recently discovered member of the innate system, the innate lymphoid cell (ILC), resides mainly in tissues. It is similar to B and T lymphocytes but differs by the absence of B- or T-cell receptors.

Monocytes and dendritic cells are derived from a common precursor in the bone marrow. When monocytes migrate into the surrounding tissue, they differentiate into macrophages, which play an important role in removing dying cells and cell debris as well as presenting antigens of ingested material for activating lymphocytes of the adaptive immune system.

2.4   Innate Immune System

Although the boundaries are fluid, a distinction is made between innate and adaptive immunity. Intruders such as fungi, spores, viruses, bacteria, amoebas, etc. can sometimes be recognized and destroyed solely by the innate immune response. This is usually achieved by pattern recognition receptors that detect conserved features of surface molecules on broad groups of microorganisms. Although the innate system does not confer long-lasting immunity, it provides an immediate initial response without which it would not be possible to survive.

Pattern Recognition by the Innate System

Receptors on cells of the innate system such as macrophages, monocytes, and neutrophils bind to two types of molecular patterns: pathogen-associated molecular patterns (PAMPs) on the surface of microbes and damage-associated molecular patterns (DAMPs) released during host cell damage or death. The detection of PAMPs is mediated by so-called toll-like receptors (TLRs) that stimulate the secretion of cytokines (see below) to activate an immune response.

A soluble mannose-binding lectin (MBL) in the blood plasma is also able to recognize a certain pattern of sugar residues on bacteria. The MBL-associated proteases trigger a cascade of complement proteins similar to the classical pathway described below, which leads to cell lysis or to phagocytosis of the bacteria (opsonization).

The Complement Cascade

About 30 different proteins constitute the complement system that straddles both the innate and the acquired immune system. It is activated via three main pathways: the classic pathway mediated by antibodies, the lectin pathway described above, and the spontaneous alternative pathway. Nine proteins of the complement system (C1–C9) are involved in the classic and lectin pathways. The first protein of the complement cascade Clq binds to the Fc part of an IgG or IgM antibody complexed with antigens (IgA, IgD, and IgE antibodies are not recognized—see next chapter for description of antibody types). The Fc-Clq complex and its associated proteases cleave the complement proteins C4 and then C2. The cascade continues until a pore-forming MAC ("membrane attack complex") of about 10 nm is formed, which consists of the polymerized C9 protein together with other proteins of the complement cascade. Water and electrolytes can now freely enter causing cell lysis. The alternative pathway is initiated by the spontaneous decay of C3 into C3a and C3b. Whereas C3b is quickly inhibited or broken down by regulatory proteins on the body's own cells, it usually remains stable on the surface of pathogenic cells. The formation of C3 convertase that cleaves C3 into C3a and C3b is at an interface of all three pathways. C3b proteins on the surface of pathogenic organisms, in addition to their function in the further cascade, can attract phagocytic cells. Other fission products in the cascade mediate an inflammatory response.

Natural Killer Cells

Natural killer cells (NK cells) of the innate immune system play an important role in the elimination of virus-infected or degenerate cells such as cancer cells. An array of activating receptors on their cell surface detect deviations on other cells and initiate a series of reactions culminating in the destruction of degenerated cells. They also secrete cytokine proteins that stimulate other immune cells such as macrophages. In common with other immune cells, they display a large number of inhibitory receptors to provide a feedback mechanism for controlling their activity.

Recognition of Self and Nonself

A major feature of NK cells is their ability to kill cells that possess low levels of MHC class 1 molecules (see following section). These molecules display peptide antigens that arise from the natural turnover and processing of proteins inside the cell. Patrolling cytotoxic T lymphocytes can distinguish between MHC1 molecules that present self or foreign and aberrant peptides from viruses and tumors. To escape surveillance, tumor cells or infected cells often downregulate the production of MHC1 molecules so that they are no longer detected by the cytotoxic T lymphocytes. However, as an important class of inhibitory receptors on NK cells exerts their inhibitory stimulus after binding to MHC1 molecules, the release from this inhibition allows the NK cells to participate in an immune attack against the aberrant cells.

2.5   Adaptive Immune System

The adaptive (or acquired) immune system requires over a week after the initial exposure to a foreign antigen before it can make an effective contribution to the immune defense. It is comprised of a multitude of lymphocytes, each of which carries a specific receptor for binding to a particular antigen. Lymphocytes having the best receptor affinity for the antigen are selected and amplified. The affinity of the receptor for the antigen can be increased by random mutations and selection of the best mutants. To achieve a more rapid response of the adaptive immune system after a renewed infection, a population of lymphocyte memory cells is established that continue to replicate for many years forming part of the first line of defense.

MHC Complex (Major Histocompatibility Complex)

The MHC complex plays a central role in the adaptive immune system. Whereas the MHC I complex is on almost every nucleated cell, the MHC II complex is mostly found on antigen-presenting cells. They are constantly loaded with peptides from the degradation of the cell's own proteins and those encoded by foreign organisms or taken up from the environment. This process is known as MHC restriction since the peptides must have a particular composition and size (8–10 amino acids for MHC 1 and 13–18 amino acids for MHC II) in order to fit into a surface groove on the MHC formed by two long α-helices flanking the peptides over a floor of β-strands. The groove in MHCI is formed by the two N-terminal domains of a heavy chain that is stabilized by a non-covalently bound ß-microglobulin subunit. In contrast, the groove in MHCII is formed by the two N-terminal domains of a heterodimer comprising α and ß subunits.

The human MHC complex is also known as the HLA (human leukocyte antigen) complex. Genes coding for the proteins of MHC are highly polymorphic. Each cell expresses six MHC class 1 alleles (HLA-A, HLA-B, and HLA-C, from each parent) and about six to eight MHC class II alleles (HLA-DP and HLA-DQ and one or two HLA-DR genes from each parent, plus different combinations). Furthermore, the human population contains hundreds of different alleles for many of these genes. It is therefore highly unlikely that any two individuals other than identical twins will express an identical MHC complex. This is a major problem for tissue transplantations since T lymphocytes recognize the peptide-binding groove of the donor MHC as a nonself antigen.

Lymphocytes

Until 1942, the main focus of immunologists was on humoral immunity. The historical adjective "humoral" refers to the humors, the extracellular body fluids. It was thought that immunological phenomena could be explained mainly by the action of antibodies. Merrill Chase, who was then working in the laboratory of Karl Landsteiner (discoverer of the ABO blood group system) on skin sensitization to particular antigens at the Rockefeller Institute, attempted to transfer the antibodies that he and Landsteiner thought were causing hypersensitivity from one guinea pig to another. They used peritoneal exudates that were clarified before injection by centrifugation. However, these experiments failed to cause any hypersensitivity to the antigen. Then in one experiment, Chase transferred an exudate that was not fully clarified, but still a little opaque, and the recipient became hypersensitive. The following experiment with fully clarified exudate was negative. He also observed that while he was able to transfer hypersensitivity with the untreated exudate, the activity disappeared after heating. In later experiments Chase was able to demonstrate that immunity to tuberculosis could be achieved by transferring white blood cells between guinea pigs. Shortly afterwards, Peter Medawar reported that circulating antibodies did not appear to play a major role in the rejection of transplants. Around 1960, James Gowan and his colleagues showed that depletion of lymphocytes in rats leads not only to a loss in the ability to reject transplants but also to a loss of the antibody response. A single cell type, the lymphocyte, was apparently responsible for both humoral and cellular immunity.

B Lymphocytes (B Cells)

Contrary to Paul Ehrlich's earlier speculations that all cells have antigen receptors, he later assumed that only specialized cells form antibodies in the blood plasma. Almost half a century later in 1948, Astrid Fagraeus reported in her doctoral thesis that plasma B cells, later shown to be the matured form of white B lymphocytes, are the cell factories that produce and secrete antibodies. Their name is derived from bursa of Fabricius, a lymphatic organ on the roof of the cloaca in birds where they were first discovered.

Initially, immature B cells in the bone marrow progress from a pro-B cell that does not express a functional B-cell receptor (BCR) to a pre-B cell that expresses the antibody heavy chain together with a surrogate light chain, which is part of the B-cell selection process. If the heavy chain has not been successfully rearranged or is otherwise flawed and cannot bind to the surrogate light chain, it is eliminated. B cells that pass this control point go on to express the usual rearranged light chain. If this is successfully accomplished, the B-cell receptor complex sends a signal that shuts down any further antibody gene rearrangements on the homologous chromosome. This process is known as allelic exclusion and ensures that only one type of heavy chain will be expressed. At this point only the IgM type of heavy chain (see next chapter) is expressed in the BCR.

The next control point is provided by self-antigens. If the BCR binds with high affinity to a cell surface antigen, the BCRs can be effectively cross-linked. This initiates a cascade of signals leading to cell death by apoptosis. Binding to a soluble antigen on the other hand results in a signal that causes the cell to become unresponsive (anergic). Yet a third possibility after high-affinity binding to an antigen is termed receptor editing. The antibody gene recombinase system is reactivated in order to replace the antigen-binding domains with domains that do not bind to the antigen. More than 90% of developing B cells in the bone marrow do not survive this selection process. The survivors migrate to the spleen where they are subjected to further negative selection with self-antigens. Those that pass this additional control point undergo further antibody gene rearrangements resulting in mature B cells expressing the IgD heavy chain immunoglobulin in addition to IgM. Some of them then localize to the marginal zone of the spleen where they specialize in detecting antigens in the circulation. The rest migrate to secondary lymphoid tissues and develop into follicular B cells that are ready to be activated with foreign antigens.

Activation of Mature B Cells

B cells can be activated by cross-linking the BCR with antigens on cell surfaces, such as some polysaccharides on bacteria. This results in a signal producing relatively low-affinity antibodies of the IgM type. In general, however, the activation of B cells is dependent on stimulation by T helper cells (see next section). The first step in this activation process is the internalization and processing by proteases of the antigens bound to the BCR, resulting in the formation of small peptides, some of which can be presented on the MHC II complex to T helper cells. When a T cell binds an MHCII complex presenting a peptide from an internalized antigen, it stimulates the activation and proliferation of the B cell. The B cells can then undergo further development in the germinal centers of the lymph node where they interact with follicular T helper cells in an environment promoting proliferation and affinity maturation of the secreted antibodies by a process of somatic hypermutation. In this process, random mutations are introduced into the antigen-binding site, and those cells expressing antibodies with higher affinities successfully compete against other cells to get the necessary signals for survival. During this process, depending on the type of cytokines secreted by the T helper cells, a so-called class switching can take place, whereby the initial IgM or IgD heavy isotypes are replaced by IgG, IgA, or IgE (see next chapter). These cells develop into antibody-producing plasma cells and memory B cells. The antibody-secreting plasma cells either remain in the lymphoid tissue or migrate to the bone marrow.

T Lymphocytes

After leaving the bone marrow, the progenitor T cells (pro-thymocytes) migrate to the thymus where they transit through the cortex into the medulla, where they eventually exit as mature T cells that then migrate to other lymphoid tissues. The maturation process, similar to that of B lymphocytes, has several control points to ensure the survival of only those T cells with correctly functioning T-cell antigen receptors, comprising two protein chains with variable antigen-binding domains analogous to the heavy and light chains of the B-cell receptor. Negative selection of T lymphocytes to remove autoreactive T cells is carried out by the medullary epithelial cells (MECs) and thymic dendritic cells. The T-cell receptors are loaded with processed peptides from proteins expressed by all of the various tissues. This is made possible by the expression of the *Aire* gene in the MECs, which codes for a transcriptional activator that facilitates the expression of proteins that would normally only be expressed in other tissues. It is estimated that more than 95% of the developing T lymphocytes do not survive the selection procedure in the thymus.

T-Cell Receptor (TCR)

The structure of the TCR is similar to the Fab fragment of an antibody (Fig. 2.2). Its α and β chains carry antigen-binding variable domains and constant domains that interact with adjacent proteins in the cell membrane comprising the TCR complex. One of the most important members of this complex is the CD3 protein cluster of γ-, δ-, ε-, and ζ-chains that provides a strong signal for T-cell activation after antigen binding. Intracellular signaling is mediated by the phosphorylation of immunoreceptor tyrosine-based activation motifs (ITAMs) that initiate the release of cytokines, such as interferon-γ (IFN-γ), interleukin-2 (IL-2), and the cytotoxic proteins perforin and granzyme. The development of a T cell to a T helper cell or to a T

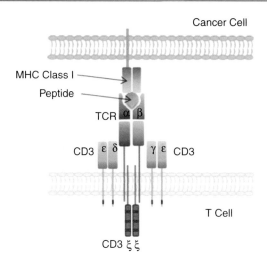

Fig. 2.2 T-cell receptor (TCR) complex. The TCR is a heterodimer comprising TCRα and TCRß flanked by a family of CD3 proteins. In this example, an MHC class I molecule presents an intracellular antigenic peptide of a cancer cell to the TCR. The CD8 co-receptor of the T cell binds to a subunit of the MHC class I molecule (not shown). (© 2019 Zhao and Cao. From Zhao L and Cao YJ. Front. Immunol. 2019; 10: 2250. Permission for use according to creative commons license (http://creativecommons.org/licenses/by/4.0/))

cytotoxic cell is thought to be influenced by the strength of the signal provided by the TCR complex and the co-receptors CD4 and CD8, one of whose expression is then terminated. After activation, CD4+ T cells differentiate and proliferate into T helper cells that produce large amounts of cytokines and the CD8+ T cells differentiate into cytotoxic T cells. (The CD nomenclature for the classification of cell surface molecules is based on a protocol originally used for identifying cluster of differentiation (CD) molecules by immunotyping with monoclonal antibodies.)

Unconventional T Cells

These T cells appear to bridge the innate and adaptive immune systems. They include cells expressing semi-invariant T-cell receptors (TCRs), such as invariant natural killer T (*i*NKT) cells and mucosal-associated invariant T (MAIT) cells. In contrast to conventional T cells which have a diverse repertoire of variable α/β chains, the invariant T cells usually have one fixed α chain variant paired with only a limited number of β chain variants. The *i*NKT cells recognize glycolipid antigen presented by CD1d, a non-polymorphic MHC class I-like molecule. MAIT cells appear to have an important function in combating microbial infections, particularly in the mucosa. They detect bacterial vitamin B metabolites presented by the MHC class I-like molecule, MR1. Another type of unconventional T cell was recently discovered that appears to recognize a cancer cell metabolite that is also presented by MR1. The powerful tool of genome-wide CRISPR-Cas9 screening was used to show that these T cells killed most human cancer types via MR1 while having no effect on non-cancerous cells. At the time of writing, the cancer-specific antigen had not been identified.

Some other T cells with diverse TCR repertoires, including intraepithelial lymphocytes (IEL) and γδT cells, share some functional features with the semi-invariant T cells. The γδT cells, representing about 2% of the total population, express a TCR that is made up of one γ (gamma) chain and one δ (delta) chain instead of the usual αβ TCR chains. The major γδT subset is represented by the chain combination Vγ9/Vδ2, which binds to an essential metabolite in the lipid biosynthesis of most pathogenic bacteria. They rapidly expand in many acute infections and may exceed the number of all other lymphocytes within a few days.

Helper T Cells

CD4+ helper T cells differentiate into five major T helper cell subsets: Th1, Th2, iT_{REG}, Th17, and T_{FH} depending on the cellular environment and the presence of specific cytokines (see below). Each of these subtypes secretes a different panel of cytokines that drive the immune response in a specific direction. Th1 cells, for example, play a major role in the body's defense against bacteria in the intracellular vesicles of macrophages, and Th2 and Th17 cells stimulate immune responses against extracellular pathogens and bacteria. iT_{REG} cells modulate the activity of other immune cells and prevent an overshooting reaction. T_{FH} cells are thought to play a primary role in the activation of B lymphocytes in lymph node follicles. After T cells bind the MHCII-peptide complex of a B cell, they release various cytokines (see below) that bind to signal-transmitting receptors. This induces B cells to develop into antibody-producing plasma cells whereby IL4, in particular, plays a major role in B-cell stimulation. The B cell then releases other cytokines, which in turn stimulate corresponding helper T cells and cytotoxic T cells. The proliferation of T cells is very much dependent on IL-2 which is secreted in large amounts by T helper cells and which stimulates autocrine receptors on the surface of both helper T cells and cytotoxic T cells. This results in a self-reinforcing humoral (soluble antibody) and cellular (cytotoxic T cell) immune response (Fig. 2.3).

Cytotoxic T Cells

After CD8+ cytotoxic T cells are activated by the presentation of antigen on the surface of professional antigen-presenting cells (APCs) in the lymph nodes, they express chemokine receptors on the cell surface which facilitate their migration to the site of an invasion by foreign organisms such as a virus. There they bind to the foreign peptide expressed by an MHC 1 complex on cells harboring the virus and form a synapse. MHCI is expressed by almost all of the body's cells and presents peptides of self and foreign proteins that have been digested in lysosomal compartments. The MHCI-peptide complexes are constantly scanned by cells of the immune

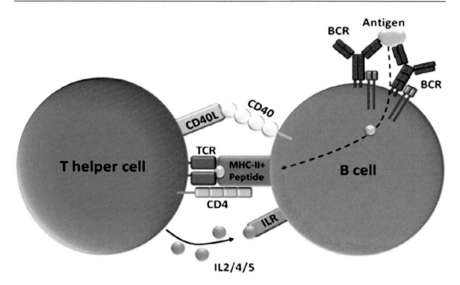

Fig. 2.3 T-cell-dependent B-cell activation. Activation of B cells after binding foreign proteins requires a first signal provided by the B-cell receptor and a second costimulatory signal provided by the interaction of CD40 with CD40L. Cytokines, particularly IL4, provide further stimulation for initiating B-cell differentiation to an antibody-producing plasma cell. (From Altaileopard (2010) according to Janeway CA et al. in Immunologie. 5. Auflage. Spektrum Akademischer Verlag, 2002)

system for their compatibility with the body's own cells. After synapse formation, perforin and granzyme are released from granular vesicles in the activated T cell. Perforin interacts with the cell membrane and facilitates the entry of granzyme into the cell interior, where it cleaves the precursor form of a caspase protease that initiates the caspase cascade resulting in apoptosis (programmed cell death). The same mechanism is used by NK cells to lyse degenerate cells.

Costimulatory Molecules

The initial activation of T and B cells requires a second signal in addition to the binding of the T- and B-cell receptors. This second signal is provided by costimulatory molecules. A major costimulatory molecule expressed on T cells is CD28 which binds to the B7 ligands CD80 (B7.1) and CD86 (B7.2) on the membrane of antigen-presenting cells. Another important costimulatory molecule is ICOS (inducible costimulatory) which binds the ligand ICOS-L. An essential costimulatory receptor for driving B-cell proliferation and differentiation is CD40. After recognizing the processed peptide of the internalized antigen presented by B cells, helper T cells, typically T_{FH} in lymph node follicles, express the CD40 ligand which binds to the B cell's CD40 receptor resulting in B-cell stimulation (Fig. 2.3). Cytokines such as IL4 secreted by the activated T helper cells provide additional stimulation to the

B cell which then undergoes cell division, antibody isotype switching (see Chap. 4), and differentiation to antibody-producing plasma cells. The need for two signals is a major mechanism for removing self-reactive cells. For example, as most of the body's cells do not present members of the B7 family on the cell surface, the lack of this signal leads to a state of anergy whereby the T cell is incapable of responding a second time to the antigen that provided the first signal.

2.6   Cytokine Signaling

The cytokines represent a broad category of small secreted glycoproteins of about 5–20 kDa in size that bind to receptors on the cell surface and initiate or strengthen an immunological response. They can be roughly divided into three categories: interleukins (signal molecules and growth factors), chemokines (initiate and direct cell migration), and interferons (antiviral agents). The term "interleukin" was originally used to describe molecules whose principal target was a leukocyte, but it is now used as a more general term for such signaling molecules. They are mainly produced by T helper cells and macrophages and influence many different processes such as initiating cell differentiation, participating in both inflammatory and anti-inflammatory responses and stimulating the production of other cytokines. They can also stimulate their own production in an autocrine fashion as mentioned above for IL-2. A high local concentration of IL-2 is maintained by signals transmitted by its own receptor on the T-cell surface that stimulates the production of more IL-2. The effect of a particular cytokine on immune cell differentiation and immune responses depends on the particular cell environment and the influence of other cytokines. In general, however, they can be roughly divided into two groups, those that enhance cellular immune responses such as TNFα and IFN-γ and those that favor antibody responses such as IL-4, IL-10, and IL-13. An overactive immune response or the administration of immunotherapeutic drugs can sometimes result in a surge of inflammatory cytokines, often described as a cytokine storm, that can have severe consequences for the patient. For example, some patients infected with SARS-CoV-2 suffered ravaging cytokine storms, and a monoclonal antibody developed to regulate the activity of T cells caused near lethal effects when first tested in humans (see Chap. 6).

2.7   Immunoregulation

To prevent the cytokine storms described above while still being able to combat pathogenic organisms, the immune response has evolved a variety of regulatory mechanisms during all stages of antigen recognition, immune cell activation, and implementation of effector functions. A simple example of a regulatory mechanism to control the amount of antibody is the negative feedback of the CD32 low-affinity receptor for IgG antibodies (FcγRII). This receptor sends a signal for the cell to downregulate antibody production after being bound by IgG-antigen complexes. Its low affinity ensures that the downregulation only occurs at high levels of IgG immune complexes. A similar mechanism exists for regulating IgE production. The low-affinity IgE receptor (FcεRII) interacts with the cell surface molecule CD21 after binding IgE-immune complexes, which then transmits a signal for downregulating the antibody production.

B-cell responses are also affected by factors that inhibit the activity of T cells, since they are dependent on T cells for their proliferation and continued activity. For example, T-cell activity can be downregulated by regulatory T cells and also by mechanisms involving specific inhibitory receptors such as CTLA-4 (CD178), PD-1 (programmed death-1, CD279), and BTLA (B- and T-lymphocyte attenuator, CD272) that render them unresponsive to antigen (anergy). Inhibitors of these so-called immune checkpoints are very much in the focus of current immunotherapeutic approaches to treat cancer since they release the brakes on T-cell activation. A more detailed description of immune checkpoints and the development of antibodies to inhibit their action is given in Chap. 6. Two other significant regulatory pathways are AICD (activation-induced cell death), which acts through the Fas receptor on activated T and B cells after binding its ligand FasL on activated T or B cells, and the activation of cell autonomous death following a lack of cytokine stimulation in the absence of antigen.

SOCS (Suppressor of Cytokine Signaling) Proteins

The predominant mechanism for the regulation of cytokine stimulation is provided by a family of SOCS proteins that are negative feedback inhibitors of the signaling cascade. The binding of the majority of cytokines to their receptors on the cell surface induces the autophosphorylation and activation of a member of the JAK (Janus kinase) family of tyrosine kinases. This kinase then phosphorylates specific tyrosines on the cytoplasmic part of the cytokine receptor which then act as docking sites for members of the signal transducers and activators of transcription (STAT) family of transcription factors. Docking facilitates the phosphorylation of the STAT by the JAK kinase, which results in its disassociation from the receptor and its translocation to the nucleus where it enhances the expression of cytokine-responsive genes including members of the SOCS family. Depending on the particular SOCS family member, negative inhibition is achieved either by binding and ubiquitination of the receptor, which initiates its degradation by the proteasome, or by blocking the active site of the JAK kinase as shown in Fig. 2.4.

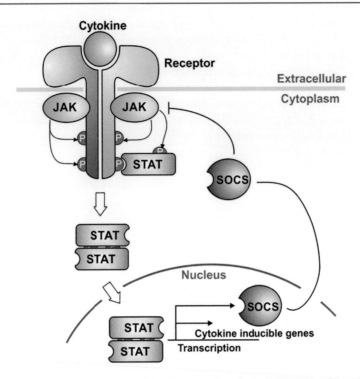

Fig. 2.4 Negative feedback inhibition of cytokine signaling via the JAK/STAT pathway. Cytokine binds to a specific receptor causing transactivation of the associated Janus kinases (JAKs). Activated JAKs then phosphorylate tyrosines on the intracellular domains of the receptor which recruit the signal transducers and activators of transcription (STAT) transcription factors. STATs are translocated into the nucleus and upregulate the transcription of cytokine-responsive genes and SOCS (suppressor of cytokine signaling) proteins which act as negative feedback inhibitors to switch off the signaling cascade. (From Morris et al. 2018. © 2018 The Protein Society. Permission from the publisher John Wiley and Sons)

Selected Literature

Crowther MD, Dolton G, Legut M, et al. Genome-wide CRISPR-Cas9 screening reveals ubiquitous T cell cancer targeting via the monomorphic MHC class I-related protein MR1 [published correction appears in Nat Immunol. 2020 Mar 2]. Nat Immunol. 2020;21(2):178–85. https://doi.org/10.1038/s41590-019-0578-8.

Delves PJ, Martin SJ, Burton DR, Roitt IM, et al. Roitt's essential immunology. 13th ed. Hoboken: Wiley; 2017.

Dimitriou ID, Clemenza L, Scotter AJ, et al. Putting out the fire: coordinated suppression of the innate and adaptive immune systems by SOCS1 and SOCS3 proteins. Immunol Rev. 2008;224:265–83. https://doi.org/10.1111/j.1600-065X.2008.00659.x.

Gallagher RB, Gilder J, Nossal GJV, Salvatore G, editors. Immunology: the making of a modern science. 1st ed. London: Harcourt Brace & Company; 1995.

Matzinger P. The danger model: a renewed sense of self. Science. 2002;296(5566):301–5. https://doi.org/10.1126/science.1071059.

Morris R, Kershaw NJ, Babon JJ. The molecular details of cytokine signaling via the JAK/STAT pathway. Protein Sci. 2018;27(12):1984–2009. https://doi.org/10.1002/pro.3519.

Murphy K, Weaver C. Janeway's immunobiology. 9th ed. New York: WW Norton & Company; 2016.

Silverstein AM. A history of immunology. 2nd ed. Amsterdam: Elsevier; 2009.

Current Approaches for Immunizing Against Cancer

3

Abstract

The discovery by Harald zur Hausen that papilloma viruses are involved in the development of cervical cancer led to the development of a vaccine based on components of the papilloma virus. This virus also appears to cause some rectal, anal, and penile cancers and 14% of head and neck cancers. The risk of developing liver cell cancers has been reduced with a vaccine against hepatitis B. In 2010, the first therapeutic vaccine, Sipuleucel-T, was approved for the treatment of advanced prostate cancer. The procedure involves isolating some of the body's own immune cells which are then incubated with tumor cell components and differentiation factors before being reintroduced into the circulation. Novel methods under development include a differential gene analysis of tumor and normal cells expressed by an individual patient followed by the injection of mRNA coding for tumor neoantigens.

3.1 Introduction

There is strong evidence that the immune system prevents various cancers from developing and metastasizing. The risk for AIDS patients with a weakened immune system after infection with HIV and for immunosuppressed patients after organ transplantation is significantly increased for a whole range of cancers. It may therefore be possible to prevent or cure some cancers by vaccination.

To prevent infections of viruses or bacteria, vaccines have been developed from inactivated viruses and bacteria or from components of the envelope or outer membrane, respectively. It may be possible to use similar procedures for those cancers caused by a virus. At least 10% of all cancers appear to be caused by a viral infection—some experts even suspect up to 20%. For those cancers not caused by viral infections, comparative analyses of normal and tumor tissues often reveal the presence of tumor neoantigens which can be used as a basis for vaccine development.

3.2   Inoculation with Immunostimulants

For more than a hundred years, inoculations have been performed with all manner of substances for stimulating the immune system to attack cancer cells. The American William Coley, for example, who is often referred to as the father of immunotherapy, injected a mixture of dead bacteria (the Coley toxins) in 1891 directly into the patient's tumor. This therapy was based on the observation that cancer patients who had suffered from a high fever after infections with such bacteria sometimes achieved a complete remission of their tumors. However, the rates of response varied widely, and the patients often suffered from serious side effects. Nevertheless, the Coley toxins were sold by the Parke-Davis Corporation from 1899 as an immunotherapeutic product for treating cancer. However, with the development of chemotherapy and radiation therapy, the drug slowly lost its importance, and production was discontinued in 1952.

Further attempts to arm the body against cancer have been made by injecting various immune-stimulating factors of the human immune system. For example, growth factors to stimulate the proliferation of immune cells and cytokines such as interleukins and interferons to prime and activate immune cells have been used in several approaches for treating cancer. However, despite the proven efficacy of some cytokines in the test tube under laboratory conditions, the clinical results were disappointing. Furthermore, since the use of such substances can cause significant side effects, they are only used for treating advanced cases of cancer in combination with chemotherapy.

3.3   Viruses and Cancer

One of the pioneers in the field of cancer viruses is the German physician Professor Harald zur Hausen. He was instrumental in discovering the link between human papillomavirus (HPV) infection and cervical cancer. As early as the nineteenth century, a physician had observed that whereas prostitutes often developed this type of cancer, nuns were not affected. Zur Hausen's hypothesis that wart viruses (papilloma viruses) are involved in the development of cervical cancer was confirmed by the isolation of HPV types 16 and 18 from the tumor cells. For his work on the development of this type of cancer, he received the Nobel Prize in Physiology or Medicine in 2008 together with the French scientists Luc Montagnier and Françoise Barré-Sinoussi for their discovery of the AIDS virus (HIV).

Vaccine Against the Papillomavirus

Based on the work of zur Hausen's research group, vaccines were developed from the capsid proteins of the virus particle (Fig. 3.1). HPV types 16 and 18 are responsible for about 70% of all cervical carcinomas, while HPV types 6 and 11 mainly contribute to the development of genital warts (condylomas). Clinical studies with

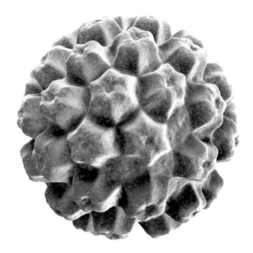

Fig. 3.1 Human papillomavirus "HPV." Infection with HPV can result in genital warts and cancer of the cervix, labia, penis, or anus as well as several other cancers. About 14% of head and neck cancers contain HPV. (Photo with the friendly permission of Sebastian Schreiter, Heidelberg)

a vaccine against HPV types 16 and 18 (Gardasil from the company Sanofi Pasteur MSD) and a vaccine against HPV types 6, 11, 16, and 18 (Cervarix from the company GlaxoSmithKline) showed a significant decrease in the expected number of cancer precursors. Since some precursors were also prevented in subjects who were infected with other types of HPV, it is likely that antibodies against the abovementioned HPV types can also recognize related viruses. To enable the production of antibodies against as many cancer-causing HPV types as possible, the company Sanofi Pasteur developed a vaccine against nine HPV types.

Despite the proven effects of the vaccine and the absence of serious side effects, the majority of young women in Germany, where the basic research leading to the development of an effective vaccine was carried out, have not been vaccinated. By comparison, in Australia where the vaccine is provided free in school-based programs, the vaccination rate is more than 80%. Relatively high vaccination rates have also been achieved in England, Holland, and Scandinavia. A significant reduction in the number of HPV infections has been registered in countries carrying out vaccination programs against HPV.

A study published by Tang and colleagues on 4433 samples of tumor tissue showed that certain types of HPV were not only associated with all cervical cancers but also with 14% of head and neck cancers. The viruses also appear to be responsible for a significant proportion of rectal, anal, and penile carcinomas. The health authorities in Australia and the United States therefore recommend vaccinating both boys and girls against HPV.

Vaccination Against Hepatitis B

At least a third of liver cell cancers appear to be caused by an infection with hepatitis B, which can be prevented by vaccination. The active substance in the vaccine is the viral surface protein HBsAg. About 35 years ago, the Taiwanese government launched a vaccination campaign against this virus, which resulted in a decrease in the number of liver cell cancers by about 50% among those vaccinated. In some countries, hepatitis C also seems to be responsible for the development of many liver cell cancers. However, as the surface proteins of this virus are constantly changing, it can escape the immune system's surveillance system.

Cell Vaccine Against a Tumor-Associated Antigen

Most vaccinations with tumor tissue extracts or isolated components of the tumor cell have so far not shown any convincing effects. One exception is the vaccine Sipuleucel-T (Provenge®), which was the first therapeutic tumor vaccine to be approved for the treatment of advanced prostate cancer. The principle of the Provenge vaccination is the administration of the body's own dendritic cells displaying tumor antigens. Dendritic cells can be found everywhere in the body and constantly scan their surroundings for the presence of foreign organisms. The foreign organisms are ingested by the dendritic cells and partially digested. Small parts of the antigen are then transported to the cell surface and presented to lymphocytes by the MHC complex (see Chap. 2), which is then bound by a matching receptor on T cells. Stimulatory signals and the release of cytokines by the dendritic cells activate T cells to attack the tumor cells.

The method used for the production of Provenge has also been used in the development of other vaccines for the therapy of various solid tumors. Basically, PBMCs (peripheral blood mononuclear cells) comprising white blood cells (approximately 60% T cells, 10% B cells, 15% natural killer cells, and 15% monocytes) are harvested from the patient by leukapheresis and shipped to the manufacturing facility. Two to 3 days later, cell fractions enriched for antigen-presenting cells (APCs) including dendritic cell precursors are obtained by two buoyant density centrifugation steps. The APCs are then incubated for 36–48 h with the tumor-associated antigen prostatic acid phosphatase (PAP) fused to granulocyte-macrophage colony-stimulating factor (GM-CSF), which appears to stimulate antigen presentation. The cells are then washed on days 3–4 before shipment back to the clinic for reinfusion into the patient. This process is repeated every 2 weeks for a complete course of three cycles.

This procedure has been modified by many research groups to achieve a better maturation of the dendritic cells and a stronger immune response. Maturation factors are now often used to mature the dendritic cell precursors prior to loading with antigen (Fig. 3.2).

The FDA approved the Sipuleucel-T vaccine in 2010 on the basis of a clinical study (the IMPACT trial) with 512 patients. The mean survival time of 21.7 months with the placebo was increased by 4.1 months, and the rate of survival after 3 years was 38% higher. Common side effects were fever, chills, fatigue, nausea, headache, and joint pain. Because individual vaccines have to be made for each patient, the cost of treatment was about $90,000 in 2010. As with many other cancer drugs, the ethical question was raised as to whether such relatively expensive treatments should be funded by national health services for an average life extension of only a

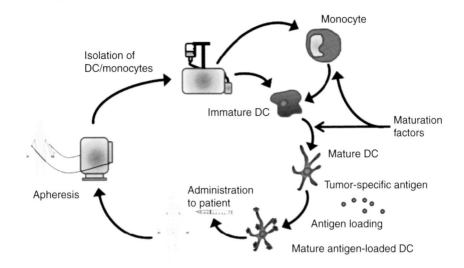

Fig. 3.2 Tumor vaccines comprising dendritic cells. Autologous dendritic cells or monocytes are obtained via an apheresis procedure. Monocytes first have to be differentiated into dendritic cells. Subsequently, dendritic cells are matured and loaded with tumor antigen. Finally, the dendritic cells are administrated to the patient. *DC* dendritic cell. (From van Willigen WW, Bloemendal M, Gerritsen WR et al. Front Immunol. 2018;9:2265. doi:https://doi.org/10.3389/fimmu.2018.02265. Permission for use according to creative commons license (http://creativecommons.org/licenses/by/4.0/))

few months. However, largely due to improved diagnostics, the survival time has been increased by 1 year for a treatment now costing $120,000, which is fairly moderate compared to the cost of a treatment with CAR-Ts (chimeric antigen receptor T cells; see Chap. 9).

As an alternative to loading DCs with tumor antigens, mRNAs can be efficiently pulsed into DCs by electroporation, which potentially results in a more persistent presentation of the tumor antigens. Many of the clinical studies testing mRNA tumor vaccines have been based on dendritic cell technology. However, the use of mRNA-based vaccines using synthetic lipid nanoparticles for delivery is steadily increasing (see below).

3.4   Nucleic Acid-Based Vaccines

For many years research efforts to develop antigen-encoding nucleic acids as vaccines were concentrated on DNA-based vectors with somewhat disappointing results. More efficient DNA vaccines such as that developed by a team of research scientists at Oxford University and AstraZeneca may be able to change this situation since their vaccine facilitates a better uptake of DNA into cells. This was accomplished by generating a modified version of the chimpanzee adenovirus ChAdOx1, which can enter cells but not replicate inside them. The result is a robust adenovirus-based vehicle comprising antigen-coding DNA that has recently been used to make a successful vaccine against the SARS-CoV-2 virus (see Chap. 2).

The instability and inefficient in vivo delivery of mRNA were regarded as major obstacles for its application as a vaccine, and some concerns were raised about its potential immunogenicity. However, these problems have been largely solved by impressive technological advances. The mRNA has been stabilized and optimized for efficient translation by modifying the cap element, 5'- and 3'-untranslated regions and the poly(A) tail. Efficient delivery systems have been devised that ensure the rapid uptake of the mRNA and its expression in the cytoplasm. Furthermore, mRNA is relatively safe since it is non-infectious and not integrated into the genome.

Two major types of mRNA have been used for making vaccines: synthetic non-replicating mRNA and self-amplifying mRNA (SAM). Most of the SAM vaccines are based on an alphavirus genome containing the genes coding for replication but in which the genes coding for the structural proteins have been replaced by a gene coding for an antigen. Immunization with SAM vaccines enables large amounts of antigen to be produced from very small doses due to its intracellular replication. However, the replicon is very large, and the production of proteins unrelated to the antigen may induce a potential host response. Furthermore, the SAM vaccines have a more complex structure than those of the relatively simple non-replicating mRNA vaccines, which are easier to manipulate.

Delivery of mRNA

A major goal of vaccines is the induction of a potent immune response by presentation of antigen to dendritic cells in the lymph nodes. It is also important that they be efficiently produced at relatively low cost, particularly when the world is confronted with a pandemic such as the present COVID-19. mRNA is itself a natural adjuvant that is recognized by the immune system as a PAMP (see Chap. 2), resulting in the stimulation of the TLR7/8 receptors on innate immune cells and the release of cytokines. However, the amplitude of this immune stimulation depends to a large extent on the composition of the delivery system.

Lipid nanoparticles (LNPs), which are somewhat similar to liposomes, are currently the most widely used delivery system for the encapsulation of mRNAs. They are primarily synthesized using (1) cationic lipids carrying tertiary or quaternary amines that associate with the polyanionic mRNA; (2) a zwitterionic lipid (e.g., 1,2-dioleoyl-*sn*-glycero-3-phosphoethanolamine (DOPE)) resembling cell membrane lipids; (3) cholesterol to stabilize the lipid bilayer, and (4) PEGylated phospholipid. The addition of PEG has become an especially important feature of LNPs since it prevents blood plasma proteins from absorbing onto the surface of the LNP, thus increasing blood circulation lifetime. It also stabilizes the LNPs, which, without added PEG, tend to fuse with one another to reduce surface tension. An overview of mRNA vaccines encapsulated in LNPs and the stimulation of an adaptive immune response against the encoded antigen is shown in Fig. 3.3.

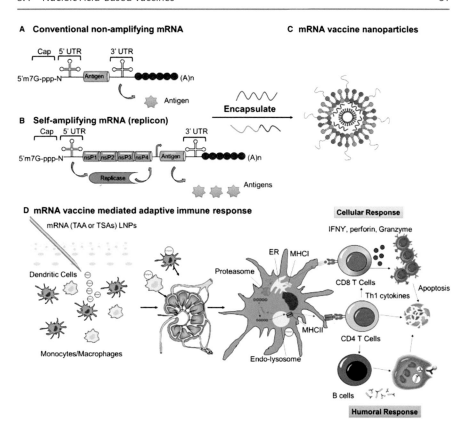

Fig. 3.3 Non-amplifying and self-amplifying mRNA vaccine and adaptive immune response. (**a**) Schematic structure of conventional non-amplifying mRNA vaccine. (**b**) Schematic structure of self-amplifying mRNA vaccine (replicon) coding for the antigen and non-structural proteins that facilitate RNA capping and replication. (**c**) Encapsulation of mRNA vaccine into lipid nanoparticles (LNPs). (**d**) The process of antigen presentation and adaptive immune activation after subcutaneous injection of mRNA vaccine LNPs. Briefly, the mRNA vaccine can be captured by antigen-presenting cells (APCs; macrophages or dendritic cells) at the injection site and transported to a draining lymph node, where mRNA is translated into protein and processed by proteasome in the APCs. Then it is presented by MHC class I or MHC class II molecules to CD8+ T cells or CD4+ T cells, thus activating both cellular and humoral responses. (From Kowalski PS et al. Mol Ther. 2019; 27(4):710–728. doi: https://doi.org/10.1016/j.ymthe.2019.02.012 with kind permission of the American Society of Gene and Cell Therapy)

In addition to this basic design for LNPs, many of the firms making mRNA vaccines have developed special features for optimizing vaccine potency. For example, BioNTech in Mainz, Germany, headed by Uğur Şahin and Özlem Türeci have developed an RNA-lipoplex (RNA-LPX) formulation that appears to be selectively taken up by dendritic cells in lymphoid compartments. Furthermore, the encoded antigen is fused to the MHC class I signal sequence and transmembrane and cytoplasmic domains for directing it to the endoplasmic reticulum, thus increasing the presentation of MHC-restricted epitopes.

The group headed by Daniel Anderson at the MIT in Cambridge, USA, screened a large complex library of lipids for optimizing both delivery to antigen-presenting cells (APCs) and the ability to provide immune stimulation via the stimulator of interferon genes (STING) pathway. Although vaccine adjuvants can stimulate an immune response, the nonspecific activation of immune pathways can result in inflammation. The researchers at MIT provided evidence that this can be avoided by specific activation of the STING pathway using the MIT lipid formulation.

The number of clinical trials with mRNA vaccines is steadily growing, and three firms in particular, CureVac (Tübingen, Germany), BioNTech (Mainz, Germany), and Moderna (Cambridge, Massachusetts, USA), have pioneered their development for the treatment and prevention of various cancers and infectious diseases.

Mutanome Engineered RNA Immunotherapy (MERIT): Personalized Therapy

The concept of the MERIT technology for the production of personalized mRNA vaccines was first put forward by the group headed by Uğur Şahin and Özlem Türeci in Mainz, Germany, in 2012. This technology is based on the discovery that of the hundreds of mutations in patient tumors, those which elicit an immunogenic response are MHC class II restricted. They can therefore stimulate CD4+ T cells and induce a potent antitumor immune response. Modern methods for high-throughput sequencing of nucleic acids from tumor biopsies facilitate the rapid identification of patient tumor-specific mutations. Several potential immunogenic candidates selected on the basis of expression and MHC class II binding prediction and restriction can then be incorporated into an mRNA vaccine. The first clinical trials using such personalized tumor vaccines are now underway. Initial studies have demonstrated robust T-cell responses, and one patient who received the vaccine in combination with anti-PD-1 therapy (see Chap. 6) was reported to have had a complete remission.

3.5   Vaccination with a Ubiquitous Tumor Marker?

As already mentioned in Chap. 2, a human T-cell clone has been isolated that is able to kill diverse cancer cell lines while having no effect on non-cancerous cells. Using genome-wide CRISPR-Cas9 screening, the T-cell receptor was shown to bind to a cancer-derived ligand presented by the monomorphic MHC class I-related protein, MR1. Once the ligand (or family of ligands) is identified, the research workers envisage the possibility of developing a universal cancer vaccine.

Selected Literature

Castle JC, Kreiter S, Diekmann J, et al. Exploiting the mutanome for tumor vaccination. Cancer Res. 2012;72(5):1081–91.

Crowther MD, Dolton G, Legut M, et al. Genome-wide CRISPR-Cas9 screening reveals ubiquitous T cell cancer targeting via the monomorphic MHC class I-related protein MR1 [published correction appears in Nat Immunol. 2020 Mar 2]. Nat Immunol. 2020;21(2):178–85. https://doi.org/10.1038/s41590-019-0578-8.

Grunwitz C, Salomon N, Vascotto F, et al. HPV16 RNA-LPX vaccine mediates complete regression of aggressively growing HPV-positive mouse tumors and establishes protective T cell memory. Onco Targets Ther. 2019;8(9):e1629259. https://doi.org/10.1080/2162402X.2019.1629259.

Hall SS. A commotion in the blood: life, death and the immune system. 1st ed. New York: Henry Holt and Co.; 1997.

Hepatitis B vaccines: WHO position paper—July 2017. Wkly Epidemiol Rec. 2017;92(27):369–92. https://apps.who.int/iris/handle/10665/255873.

Kantoff PW, Higano CS, Shore ND, et al. Sipuleucel-T immunotherapy for castration-resistant prostate cancer. N Engl J Med. 2010;363(5):411–22. https://doi.org/10.1056/NEJMoa1001294.

Kash N, Lee MA, Kollipara R, et al. Safety and efficacy data on vaccines and immunization to human papillomavirus. J Clin Med. 2015;4:614–33. https://doi.org/10.3390/jcm4040614.

Kowalski PS, Rudra A, Miao L, Anderson DG. Delivering the messenger: advances in technologies for therapeutic mRNA delivery. Mol Ther. 2019;27(4):710–28. https://doi.org/10.1016/j.ymthe.2019.02.012.

Kreiter S, Vormehr M, van de Roemer N, et al. Mutant MHC class II epitopes drive therapeutic immune responses to cancer. Nature. 2015;520:692–6.

Miao L, Li L, Huang Y, et al. Delivery of mRNA vaccines with heterocyclic lipids increases anti-tumor efficacy by STING-mediated immune cell activation. Nat Biotechnol. 2019;37(10):1174–85. https://doi.org/10.1038/s41587-019-0247-3.

Peng M, Mo Y, Wang Y, et al. Neoantigen vaccine: an emerging tumor immunotherapy. Mol Cancer. 2019;18:128. https://doi.org/10.1186/s12943-019-1055-6.

Sahin U, Derhovanessian E, Türeci Ö, et al. Personalized RNA mutanome vaccines mobilize polyspecific therapeutic immunity against cancer. Nature. 2017;547:222–6.

Tang KW, Alaei-Mahabadi B, Samuelsson T, et al. The landscape of viral expression and host gene fusion and adaptation in human cancer. Nat Commun. 2013;4:2513. https://doi.org/10.1038/ncomms3513.

van Willigen WW, Bloemendal M, Gerritsen WR, et al. Dendritic cell cancer therapy: vaccinating the right patient at the right time. Front Immunol. 2018;9:2265. https://doi.org/10.3389/fimmu.2018.02265.

Generation, Structure, and Function of Antibodies

4

Abstract

The major role of antibodies is to target foreign bodies for the artillery of the immune system. Binding sites for antigens are located in the variable regions at the end of the two arms of the Y-shaped antibody, and binding sites for components of the immune system are located in the constant regions of the basal Fc domain. There are five classes of constant regions (A, D, E, G, and M) which determine the particular function of an antibody. The immune system has evolved a highly sophisticated system of antibody gene rearrangements involving DNA-binding proteins, a nuclease, a nucleotide transferase, a protein kinase, a ligase, exonucleases, and polymerases. Antibody diversity is created by a random rearrangement of genes coding for various sections of the antibody variable domain and also by the random addition or removal of nucleotides during the processes of DNA cleavage and ligation. Further diversity is created after an antigen binds to a B lymphocyte in the germinal centers. This stimulates B-cell proliferation and initiates a system for introducing a high number of mutations (somatic hypermutation) into the DNA region coding for the antigen-binding CDRs (complementarity-determining regions). B cells carrying receptors with an enhanced ability to bind antigens are then positively selected for further expansion. The antibody structure is further stabilized by posttranslational glycosylation of the Fc domain. Modifications of the oligosaccharide structure can enhance antibody effector functions which are located in the same part of the molecule.

4.1   Introduction

Before 1955 it was a mystery how the human body could contain such an enormous diversity of antibodies. One hypothesis was that an antigen (*anti*body *gen*erating) somehow impressed its shape onto a cell thereby inducing it to synthesize an antibody with the corresponding specificity. In 1955, Niels Jerne published a "selective" hypothesis for the selection and amplification of an antigen-binding antibody from a large set of different antibodies. He imagined that an antigen after injection formed a complex with a natural antibody. The complex was then taken up by a macrophage in which the antibody acted as a template for synthesizing more antibodies. In 1957, David Talmage proposed that the concept would make more sense if the unit of selection was a cell with an antibody on its surface. In the same year, Frank MacFarlane Burnet elucidated his groundbreaking clonal selection theory for the regulation and amplification of specific antibodies. Burnet proposed that each lymphocyte displays a specific immunoglobulin that will later be synthesized once the cell is stimulated to proliferate and differentiate by the binding of a complementary antigen. His theory also included the concept of clonal deletion, which explained the findings reported by Peter Medawar in 1953 that exposure to foreign tissues during embryonic development resulted in tolerance. The stage was finally set for rapid advances in the field of cellular immunology when the work of James Gowan in the early 1960s showed that the removal of small lymphocytes from rats resulted in the loss of the adaptive immune response (see Chap. 2).

4.2   Elucidation of the Antibody Structure

In 1962, Rodney Porter showed that three large antibody fragments (Fab′, Fab′2, and Fc) were obtained after digestion with the enzymes pepsin and papain, which indicated a "Y"-shaped molecule (Fig. 4.1). Two heavy chains are connected to

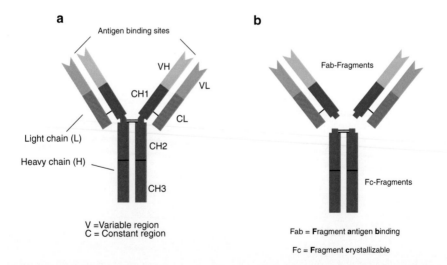

Fig. 4.1 Structure of an IgG antibody. (**a**) Structure of an IgG antibody with variable domains that contain binding sites for antigens and constant domains that contain binding sites for components of the immune system. (**b**) Characteristic Fab′ and Fc fragments after digestion with papain. Only the Fab′ fragments still bind antigen. *V* variable region, *C* constant region, *Fab* fragment antigen binding, *Fc* fragment crystallizable

each other and to two light chains by disulfide bridges. The disulfide bridges between the heavy chains form a flexible hinge region. A major problem for clarifying the primary structure was the heterogeneity of the antibodies, since each antibody contains unique sequences in the variable regions. A discovery by Bence Jones in 1865 provided the solution. He had discovered large amounts of a homogeneous protein in the urine of certain cancer patients. It is now known that such patients suffer from multiple myeloma, which arises from a single antibody-producing plasma cell. The Bence Jones proteins were identical to the light chains of immunoglobulins. Several such proteins were sequenced by Norbert Hilschmann in 1965, who found that the chains consisted of constant and variable domains. Gerald Edelman then succeeded in 1969 in sequencing a complete antibody obtained from murine myeloma cells. With a length of 1300 amino acids, it was the longest protein to have been sequenced at that time. Edelman and Porter won the Nobel Prize in Physiology or Medicine in 1972 for their work on elucidating the antibody structure. The three-dimensional structure of a monoclonal antibody was elucidated by Alexander McPherson in 1982.

4.3   Antibody Diversity

For many years immunologists and geneticists were divided as to whether antibody diversity resided in the germline sequence or whether antibody diversity was somehow generated during development. In 1965 Dreyer and Bennett had suggested that one of many V genes may be excised from the genome and somehow joined to the single C gene. It wasn't until the early 1970s that techniques evolved, such as the purification of specific eukaryotic mRNAs, which enabled the phenomenon of antibody diversity to be investigated. Using the newly discovered restriction enzymes and DNA fractionation by electrophoresis, Susumu Tonegawa was able to demonstrate that the patterns of hybridization with "V plus C" and "C" probes from a light chain mRNA to fractionated germline DNA (from embryos) and to κ-myeloma DNA were quite different. Indeed, they were consistent with the occurrence of separate V and C genes and a joined V plus C gene. Tonegawa then went on to play a leading role in the application of recombinant DNA technology developed in the 1970s to demonstrate how random rearrangements and mutations of the immunoglobulins could generate millions of different antibody specificities, for which he was awarded a Nobel Prize in Physiology or Medicine in 1987 as the sole recipient.

4.4   Antibody Gene Rearrangement

The human body contains approximately 10^{10} to 10^{12} B lymphocytes. However, the number of circulating peripheral naïve mature B cells is estimated to be about 10^9, a number that is far less than the potential antibody diversity. The antibody heavy chain variable regions arise from the rearrangement and junctional diversification of about 43 functional V gene segments, 23 D gene segments, and 6 J gene segments.

The antibody kappa and lambda light chain variable regions are rearrangements of approximately 36 and 32 V gene segments, respectively, each combined with one of five corresponding J gene segments (Fig. 4.2).

The agents and mechanism of antibody diversification are briefly as follows:

- **RAG 1** and **RAG 2**: *r*ecombination-*a*ctivating *g*ene proteins bind to specific recombination signal sequences (**RSS**) flanking the antibody gene segments.
- **RSS**: conserved heptamer and nanomer sequences separated by a spacer which is either 12 bp (flanking D gene segments) or 23 bp (flanking V and J gene segments), which correspond approximately to one or two turns of the DNA helix, respectively. The RAG proteins form a recombinase complex with other DNA-binding proteins which only permits recombination between recombination signals with 12 and 23 base pair spacers (the 12/23 rule). This allows the joining of

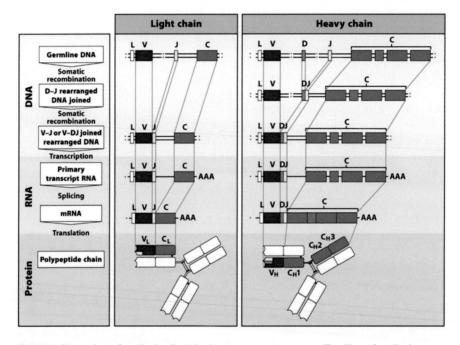

Fig. 4.2 Generation of antibody diversity by gene rearrangements. Families of antibody genes coding for V, D, and J domains (heavy chain) and V and J domains (light chain), respectively, are randomly combined with one another as shown above. For generation of the light chain variable domain, one of the 44κ or 38λ V genes is ligated with one of the five J genes. For generation of the heavy chain variable domain, 1 of the 23 D genes is ligated with 1 of the 6 J genes, followed by the ligation of the DJ fusion gene with 1 of the approximately 43 functional V genes. Further diversity is created by the random addition and removal of nucleotides at the ends of the gene segments during ligation. The variable domain gene is first fused with IgM or IgD constant domains. After activation by antigen in the germinal centers, the constant domains are replaced with those of IgG, IgA, or IgE, and further diversity is created by somatic hypermutation. (From Janeway's Immunobiology 7E by Kenneth Murphy and Paul Travers Mark Walport. © 2008 by Garland Science, Taylor & Francis Group, LLC. Used by permission of W.W. Norton & Company, Inc.)

D gene segments to both V and J gene segments but ensures that V gene segments will not directly combine with J gene segments.

- **Recombinase Complex**: Besides the RAG proteins, other key enzymes involved are terminal deoxynucleotidyl transferase (TdT), the Artemis nuclease, a member of the ubiquitous "non-homologous end joining" (NHEJ) pathway for DNA repair and the DNA-dependent protein kinase (DNA-PK) as well as a ligase and polymerases.
- **Process**: The RAG proteins make single-strand nicks between the first base of the RSS and the coding segment resulting in a hairpin on the coding segment and a blunt end on the signal segment. DNA-PK binds to each broken DNA end and recruits the enzymes shown above. A key step is the opening of the hairpin by Artemis. TdT adds random nucleotides to one strand in a 5′ to 3′ direction. Lastly, exonucleases can remove nucleotides from the coding ends, and polymerases insert nucleotides to make the two ends compatible for joining. The coding ends are then ligated together by a DNA ligase. The random addition and removal of nucleotides greatly increases antibody diversity (Fig. 4.3).

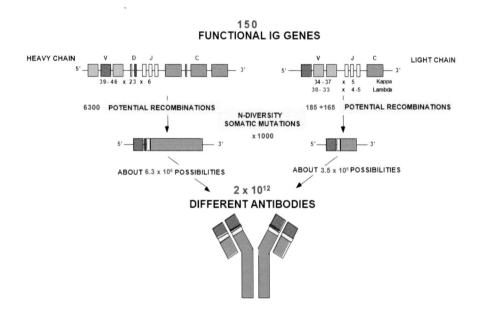

Fig. 4.3 Approximate potential size of naïve antibody libraries in humans. The mechanisms of diversity that occur at the DNA level in the B cell result in about 6.3×10^6 and 3.5×10^6 different heavy and light chains, respectively, and the pairing of one heavy chain with one light chain results in a potential repertoire of 2×10^{12} different antibodies. Disulfide bridges are not shown. The gene regions involved in the H chain V-D-J and L chain V-J rearrangements are highlighted: *V* dark green, *D* red, *J* yellow. (Lefranc M-P, Lefranc G. Biomedicines. 2020; 8(9): 319. https://doi.org/10.3390/biomedicines8090319. With permission of M-P. Lefranc and G. Lefranc, LIGM, Founders and Authors of IMGT®, the international ImMunoGeneTics information system®, http://www.imgt.org)

4.5   Somatic Hypermutation (SHM)

When an antigen binds to the antibody receptor on the surface of a B cell in the germinal centers of secondary lymphoid organs, it is stimulated to proliferate. At the same time, the B-cell receptor locus undergoes a very high mutation rate at regions concentrated in those parts of the DNA corresponding to the complementarity-determining regions (CDRs) of the antibody's variable domains. The CDRs largely determine the antigen specificity and binding affinity. One of the enzymes involved in this process is the activation-induced cytidine deaminase (AID) that deaminates cytosine to uracil in DNA.

It was previously thought that SHM could be explained by a repair enzyme removing uracils and insertion of mutations by error-prone DNA polymerases. However, the most plausible mechanism that explains all the present data according to Steele (2017) is based on the error-prone reverse transcription of the base-modified pre-mRNA by DNA polymerase η. Ig pre-mRNA is copied off the transcribed DNA strand carrying prior AID C-to-U deamination lesions. It also accumulates mutations arising from "adenosine deaminases acting on RNA" (ADARs) which edit A-to-I modifications. This already base-modified pre-mRNA sequence is then copied back to the B-lymphocyte genomic DNA and integrated at the rearranged V[D]J site. During the proliferation process, many different mutants are expressed, thus allowing the positive clonal selection of those B cells carrying receptors with an enhanced ability to bind antigens.

4.6   Class Switch Recombination (CSR)

Naïve mature B lymphocytes produce both IgM and IgD antibodies. Their constant domains are coded by the first two constant domain DNAs in the immunoglobulin locus. After activation in the germinal centers by antigen binding, these constant domains can be replaced by one of the five IgG families or IgA or IgE. The switching process is carried out by removing a portion of the heavy chain gene locus and rejoining the ends using many of the enzymes that also play a role in somatic hypermutation. The type of heavy chain chosen by CSR depends on the reception of various signals mediated by helper T cells (see Chap. 2). These signaling patterns have evolved to induce the expression of the most appropriate heavy chain constant domain for combating a particular foreign organism.

4.7   Role of Antibodies

The first antibody preparation for the treatment of an infectious disease was a neutralizing serum from a horse immunized against diphtheria toxin (see Chap. 1). The neutralizing or blocking effect of antibodies is also used by modern cancer immunotherapies. For example, therapeutic antibodies can neutralize essential growth factors or block access to their receptors on the cell surface. If the growth signals are prevented from binding to their receptors on the cell surface, growth stagnates and the tumor cell dies. More recently, antibodies have been used to block the access of inhibitory ligands to immune checkpoints (see Chap. 6).

The major role of antibodies in immune defense is to mark foreign bodies for attack by the artillery of the immune system. Cytotoxic natural killer (NK) cells, for example, express receptors on their cell surface for binding to specific epitopes on the antibody Fc domain. After binding, the receptors send stimulatory signals to initiate ADCC (antibody-dependent cellular cytotoxicity, Chap. 6). The antibody constant domains can also bind and activate C1 complement, which initiates the complement cascade resulting in CDC (complement-dependent cytotoxicity). Other examples are given below.

4.8   Binding Sites for Antibody Fc Domains

– Fc receptors on phagocytes (macrophages and neutrophils): microorganisms such as bacteria are enveloped and destroyed (phagocytosis).
– Fc receptors on natural killer cells: NK cells attack infected and degenerate cells such as tumor cells. The release of the enzyme granzyme B from the NK cell through pores in the target cell triggers a cascade of other enzymes (the caspases), which leads to the breakdown of the cell (apoptosis). This process is known as antibody-dependent cellular cytotoxicity (ADCC).
– Fc receptors on mast cells: the release of histamine leads to inflammation. Inflammatory factors that both attract other immune cells and cause dilation of the blood vessels play an important role in combating intruders such as bacteria.
– Clq (the first protein of the complement cascade): binding of IgM or IgG complexed with antigens to Clq initiates the complement cascade leading to the production of the pro-inflammatory C3a and C5a and to the formation of a MAC complex (membrane attack complex) consisting of C5b, C6, C7, C8, and polymeric C9 complement proteins, which can induce cell lysis by complement-dependent cytotoxicity (CDC).

4.9   IgG Fc Receptors (FcγR)

Most therapeutic antibodies are of the IgG type, which is the most abundant in serum. IgG antibodies have binding sites on the second constant domain of the heavy chain (CH2) for receptors on all of the cells of the immune system except T cells. The major groups of FcγR are the activating receptors FcγRI, FcγRIIa, and FcγRIIIa, the inhibitory receptor FcγRIIb, and the glycosylphosphatidylinositol (GPI)-anchored FcγRIIIb. Activating FcγRs contain an intracellular immunoreceptor tyrosine-based activation motif (ITAM) for signal transduction. The tyrosine residues within this motif become phosphorylated by the Src family of kinases after the receptor is bound by antibodies. The phosphorylated tyrosines serve as docking sites for other proteins involved in the signaling cascade of cell activation. The inhibitory FcγRIIb, on the other hand, carries an immunoreceptor tyrosine-based inhibitory motif (ITIM) that inhibits the signaling pathway (see Chap. 2). The activating receptor FcγRIIIa is highly expressed on NK cells, which appear to be the most potent immune cells for ADCC.

4.10 Classes of Immunoglobulins

An overview of the major classes of antibody is shown in Fig. 4.4.
Occurrence and function of immunoglobulin classes:

– IgG (monomer): its five subclasses (IgG1, IgG2, IgG3, IgG4, and IgG, named according to their frequency in serum) account for approx. 80% of all antibodies; only IgG can cross the placenta to protect the child from infection for a few months after birth.
– IgE (monomer): less than 0.1% of the antibodies; only bound by receptors on the surface of mast cells, which play an important role in allergies and fighting parasitic infestations.
– IgD (monomer): less than 0.2% of the antibodies; involved in the activation of B lymphocytes.
– IgA (dimer): its two subclasses account for 10–15% of the antibodies; can be transported through epithelia (e.g., the inner lining of the intestinal tract); first

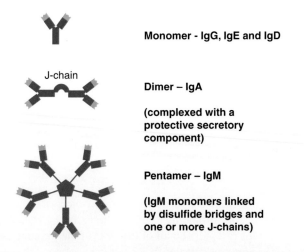

Monomer - IgG, IgE and IgD

Dimer – IgA

(complexed with a protective secretory component)

Pentamer – IgM

(IgM monomers linked by disulfide bridges and one or more J-chains)

Fig. 4.4 Antibody classes. The five subclasses of IgGs are the most abundant and can cross the placenta; IgEs play a major role in allergies and fighting parasite infestation; IgDs play a role in the activation of B cells; the two subclasses of IgA are secreted by mucous membranes and play an essential role in the first line of defense. They are also secreted into milk. Mainly dimeric (joined by a J chain), they are also complexed with a secretory component that protects them, for example, against proteolytic digestion in the gastrointestinal tract; IgMs are the first antibodies produced after an infection. IgG, IgD, and IgE have three constant domains; IgE and IgM have four constant domains

immune defense on the mucous membranes of the mouth and gastrointestinal tract; only antibody in milk.
– IgM (pentamer): 5–10% of the antibodies; first antibodies produced after infection; the five antigen-binding sites of the pentamer facilitate agglutination and phagocytosis of bacteria.

In contrast to IgG, IgD, and IgA antibodies, which contain three constant domains, IgM and IgE antibodies have an additional fourth domain.

The determination of the Ig type is important for the treatment of a suspected infection. For example, in the case of a suspected toxoplasmosis infection during pregnancy, a high IgG titer with only a little IgM indicates a previous infection. A high IgM titer indicates a current infection that needs to be treated. IgM antibodies are detectable 1 week after infection and reach maximum values after 2–4 weeks. IgG antibodies appear later and reach maximum values after about 2–4 months.

4.11 Long Half-Life of IgG Antibodies

The ability of IgG as the only class of antibody to cross the placenta is due to its binding site for the neonatal receptor (FcRn) on the cell membranes of the placenta. This receptor is also present on the surface of the endothelium (inner cell layer on the inside of blood vessels). Antibodies are continuously internalized into small cellular transport vesicles (pinocytosis), which fuse with larger vesicles (endosomes) inside the cell. Normally, serum proteins are transported further to the lysosomes where they are degraded. However, at the relatively low pH (<pH 6.5) of the endosome, IgG antibodies bind very tightly to the membrane-bound FcRn and are transported back to the cell surface in small vesicles that bud off from the endosome. At the higher pH on the cell surface, the IgG no longer tightly bind to FcRn and are released into the bloodstream. An IgG antibody therefore has a significantly longer half-life than other antibody classes. Its half-life is 20–25 days compared to only 6 days for IgA, 5 days for IgM, 2–8 days for IgD, and 1–5 days for IgE (according to Segen's Medical Dictionary). The half-life of a therapeutic antibody is always measured to determine an optimal dosage.

4.12 Antibody Glycosylation

IgG antibodies, which account for nearly all of the therapeutic antibodies approved for clinical use, are glycosylated on a conserved asparagine residue at position 297 (Asn-297) on the CH2 subunit in the Fc domain. The oligosaccharide plays an essential role both in the stability of the CH2 domain and in the modulation of the antibody effector functions. Deglycosylated antibodies are thermally less stable and more prone to unfolding and degradation. The process of glycosylation starts in the endoplasmic reticulum (ER) with the transfer of a pre-formed lipid-linked glycan comprising two *N*-acetylglucosamines (GlcNAc) followed by nine branched

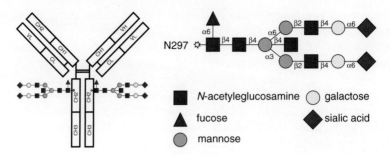

Fig. 4.5 Structure of a fully processed IgG-Fc *N*-glycan. The asparagine 297-linked glycan is located within the CH2 domains of the Fc fragment and consists of a complex, biantennary structure. In vivo, such a fully processed glycan will be found only in trace amounts as the majority of antibodies will carry either no, one, or two galactose residues, and only a fraction of those carrying galactose will additionally possess sialic acid. (Reprinted by permission of Springer Nature from Quast I, Peschke B, Lünemann JD. Cell Mol Life Sci (2017) **74**, 837-847. doi: https://doi.org/10.1007/s00018-016-2366-z)

mannose (Man) residues and three glucose (Glc) residues to an asparagine residue at position 297 of the heavy chain amino acid sequence. This structure is highly conserved in eukaryotes and serves as a quality control marker for correct folding of proteins carrying *N*-glycans. The antibody is then transferred to the Golgi where it can be fully processed to the glycosylated IgG shown in Fig. 4.5. However, this fully processed form only occurs in small amounts in vivo where one or both of the galactose residues are usually missing. In addition to the Fc *N*-glycan, about 15–20% of the IgG antibodies in serum are glycosylated in the variable domains, which may have some impact on antigen binding.

The binding sites for CDC and ADCC (see above) are fairly close to the Asn-297 on the CH2 domain. Modification of the oligosaccharide can therefore have an impact on both of these effector functions as well as on antibody pharmacodynamics (PD) and pharmacokinetics (PK). For example, the removal of fucose from the Fc *N*-glycan increases the binding affinity of IgGs to the FcγRIIIA (CD16A) receptor on natural killer cells which can result in a significant increase in the efficacy of cell killing by ADCC.

4.13   Chain Folding of an Antibody

Each variable and constant domain of the antibody heavy and light chains consists of a chain of amino acids, which—like a new shoelace before use—is folded several times on itself. The two opposite ends of the shoelace connect each domain with the two neighboring domains. Figure 4.6a shows the folding of the amino acid chain in an antibody with 12 domains (IgE and IgM antibodies have an extra additional constant domain, CH4). Interchain disulfide bonds at the base of the CH1-CL domains and in the hinge region between the heavy chains as well as intrachain disulfide

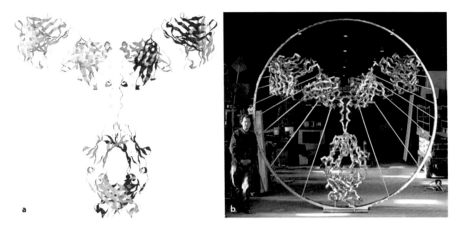

Fig. 4.6 Chain folding of an antibody. The pleated sheet structure is based on a model by Eduardo Padlan (**a**), which was used as the inspiration for the sculpture *Angel of the West* by Julian Voss-Andreae (**b**). To emphasize the similarity to the proportions of the human body, the model of the antibody is shown in a ring reflecting that of the Vitruvian Man drawn by Leonardo da Vinci (© Julian Voss-Andreae, with kind permission)

bonds in each domain serve to stabilize the antibody structure. Alluding to the similarity of the antibody structure with the human body in the drawing of the Vitruvian Man by Leonardo da Vinci, Julian Voss-Andreae created the IgG sculpture *Angel of the West* shown in Fig. 4.6b.

4.14 Antibody Terminology

The INN (international nonproprietary name) for mAbs named before 2017 had four components: (1) the prefix for the given name; (2) the target organ (e.g., tumor); (3) the origin of the antibody; and (4) the suffix "mab." Examples of the target organ are tu/t, tumor; li/l, immune system; ci/c, cardiovascular system; and ne/n, neurons. The vowel is not used when a second follows. Before 2009, three letters were sometimes used for the target organ (e.g., lim instead of li/l). The origin of the antibody before 2017 was denoted by the following endings: omab, mouse; imab, primates; ximab, chimeric; zumab, humanized; and umab, human. Some examples of pre-2017 antibody names are rituximab, Ri (given name)/tu (tumor)/ximab (chimeric); trastuzumab, Tras (given name)/tu (tumor)/zumab (humanized); and nivolumab, Nivo (given name)/l (immune system)/umab (human). From 2014 to 2017, the antibody's origin was determined using a sequence alignment procedure, whereby the -xi or -zu infix was determined solely by the alignment of the V genes. This led to inconsistent source designations, and the WHO decided to drop the infix denoting the origin in 2017. Regarding mAbs against tumor targets, the infix t(u) was changed to ta (tumor antigen).

Selected Literature

Boune S, Hu P, Epstein AL, Khawli LA. Principles of N-linked glycosylation variations of IgG-based therapeutics: pharmacokinetic and functional considerations. Antibodies. 2020;9:22. https://doi.org/10.3390/antib9020022.

Chiu ML, Goulet DR, Teplyakov A, Gilliland GL. Antibody structure and function: the basis for engineering therapeutics. Antibodies. 2019;8(4):55. https://doi.org/10.3390/antib8040055.

Delves PJ, Martin SJ, Burton DR, Roitt IM, et al. Roitt's essential immunology. 13th ed. Hoboken: Wiley; 2017.

Gallagher RB, Gilder J, Nossal GJV, Salvatore G, editors. Immunology: the making of a modern science. 1st ed. London: Harcourt Brace & Company; 1995.

Inbar D, Hochman J, Givol D. Localization of antibody-combining sites within the variable portions of heavy and light chains. Proc Natl Acad Sci U S A. 1972;69(9):2659–62. https://doi.org/10.1073/pnas.69.9.2659.

Lefranc M-P, Lefranc G. Immunoglobulins or antibodies: IMGT® bridging genes, structures and functions. Biomedicine. 2020;8(9):319. https://doi.org/10.3390/biomedicines8090319.

Murphy K, Weaver C. Janeway's immunobiology. 9th ed. New York: WW Norton & Company; 2016.

Narciso JET, Uy IDC, Cabang AB, et al. Analysis of the antibody structure based on high-resolution crystallographic studies. New Biotechnol. 2011;28(5):435–47. https://doi.org/10.1016/j.nbt.2011.03.012.

Padlan EA. Anatomy of the antibody molecule. Mol Immunol. 1994;31:169–217. https://doi.org/10.1016/0161-5890(94)90001-9.

Parrena PWHI, Carter PJ, Plückthun A. Changes to international nonproprietary names for antibody therapeutics 2017 and beyond: of mice, men and more. MAbs. 2017;9(6):898–906. https://doi.org/10.1080/19420862.2017.1341029.

Quast I, Peschke B, Lünemann JD. Regulation of antibody effector functions through IgG Fc N-glycosylation. Cell Mol Life Sci. 2017;74:837–47. https://doi.org/10.1007/s00018-016-2366-z.

Rees AR. Understanding the human antibody repertoire. MAbs. 2020;12(1):1729683. https://doi.org/10.1080/19420862.2020.1729683.

Segen JC. Concise Dictionary of Modern Medicine. McGraw-Hill Companies, Inc.; 2006.

Silverstein AM. A history of immunology. 2nd ed. Amsterdam: Elsevier; 2009.

Steele EJ. Reverse transcriptase mechanism of somatic hypermutation: 60 years of clonal selection theory. Front Immunol. 2017;8:1611. https://doi.org/10.3389/fimmu.2017.01611.

Umaña P, Jean-Mairet J, Moudry R, et al. Engineered glycoforms of an antineuroblastoma IgG1 with optimized antibody-dependent cellular cytotoxic activity. Nat Biotechnol. 1999;17(2):176–80. https://doi.org/10.1038/6179.

Of Mice and Men: Production of Therapeutic Antibodies

5

Abstract

In 1975, Georges Köhler and César Milstein discovered a method for producing larger quantities of identical (monoclonal) antibodies. They fused a B cell from the spleen of an immunized mouse with a myeloma tumor cell. The result was an immortal hybridoma cell that produced abundant monoclonal antibodies. For therapeutic use, the immunogenicity of monoclonal antibodies has been reduced either by replacing the murine constant domains with human sequences (chimeric mAbs) or by replacing all of the non-binding parts of the antibody with human sequences (humanized mAbs). Completely human antibodies have been produced using transgenic mice in which the murine antibody genes have been replaced by human genes. To obtain human antibodies in vitro without immunization, large antibody libraries have been created using genetic engineering methods that mimic to some extent the in vivo generation of antibodies. To screen these enormous libraries, the clonal selection system of the immune system was also imitated by coupling the antibody gene with its antibody product expressed on the surface of a microorganism, usually a bacteriophage. Those microorganisms were selected that bound with the highest affinity to immobilized antigens. The antibody genes could then be transfected into a eukaryotic cell line (usually CHO cells) to produce sufficient quantities of a therapeutic antibody.

5.1 Introduction

The scientific journey of discovery resulting in the large-scale production of antibodies with a unique specificity for a particular antigen can be traced back to the arrival of the Argentinian César Milstein at the Laboratory of Molecular Biology in Cambridge in 1963, the same laboratory where Francis Crick and James Watson solved the structure of DNA in 1953. He was invited to come by the head of the Protein Chemistry division, Frederick Sanger, who had collaborated with Milstein on a project a few years earlier and who had heard of Milstein's problems after the military coup in Argentina in 1962. The military regime was persecuting political dissenters, and Jews like César Milstein were regarded as being associated with the communists.

5.2   Myeloma Cell Cultures

At the Laboratory of Molecular Biology, Milstein became interested in the structure of antibodies and their enormous diversity. A major discovery by Henry Kunkel in 1951, an immunologist at the Rockefeller Institute in New York, provided a major tool for Milstein's research. Kunkel had observed that malignant plasma cells of patients with multiple myeloma produced just one kind of antibody. Various myeloma cell lines became available after 1962 due to an unexpected finding by Michael Potter that an injection of mineral oil into the peritoneal cavity of BALB/c mice induced the growth of myeloma cells, which were later adapted to be grown in tissue culture.

5.3   Fused Myeloma Cell Lines

In 1966, Sydney Brenner and César Milstein proposed that antibody diversity was the result of somatic mutation. To provide evidence for this hypothesis, Milstein studied the mutations arising in cloned myeloma cells in soft agar, a technique used in his laboratory by the Australian post doc Dick Cotton. One of Cotton's objectives was to study why only one set of parental genes were used to produce an antibody, a process known as allelic exclusion. By fusing two myeloma cell lines using inactivated Sendai virus, Cotton and Milstein wanted to see which genes would be silenced and what the effect of fusion would have on the antibody structure. Surprisingly, they found that a hybridoma of a rat myeloma cell with a murine myeloma cell produced both parental antibodies; there was no allelic exclusion and no antibody gene scrambling. They therefore theorized that these processes occurred early in cell differentiation. Milstein presented these and further results on myeloma fusions at the Basel Institute for Immunology in 1973. In the audience was George Köhler, on temporary leave from the University of Freiburg while completing his doctoral thesis. Köhler took an instant liking to Milstein and asked to join him in Cambridge, where he started work in 1974.

5.4   First Hybridoma

To make further progress on understanding the molecular basis of antibody specificity, Milstein and Köhler needed a cell line producing an antibody with a clearly defined specificity. Some scientists had, in fact, already devised ways to make antibodies with known specificities. For example, Joseph Sinkovics, a Hungarian scientist working on viral mouse leukemia at the M.D. Anderson Hospital and Tumor Institute in Texas, became interested in a mouse lymphoma cell line with virus-like particles on its surface that induced an immune response. In 1968, he succeeded in growing the cells in tissue culture by co-incubation with spleen cells from mice that had rejected the lymphoma cells. Surprisingly, new cells appeared that produced not only virus particles but also specific antibodies against the virus. He hypothesized that this was the result of a natural fusion between a splenic plasma cell with an immortalizing mouse lymphoma cell. Such hybrid cells were later named hybridomas. Unfortunately, Sinkovics had to abandon further work on this project because the National Cancer Institute (NCI) refused funding on the grounds that although scientifically sound it could not envisage any therapeutic applications for the antibodies.

5.5   Cloned B Lymphocytes

Another method for generating monoclonal antibodies was pursued by the team of Brigitte Ita Askonas at the National Institute for Medical Research which succeeded in cloning B lymphocytes in genetically identical irradiated mice. However, the clones could only be maintained for 6 months. Norman Klinman at the University of Pennsylvania devised a sophisticated technique employing irradiated mice that were injected with antibody-producing cells. Cultures of spleen cells incubated with antigen were able to produce monoclonal antibodies, but the cells only survived for a maximum of 3 months. A more promising avenue of research was opened up by Jerrold Schwaber and Edward Cohen at the University of Chicago in 1973. They succeeded in fusing human B lymphocytes with mouse myeloma cells. The hybrid cell produced both antibodies from the myeloma cell line and antibodies from the lymphocyte. However, the cells did not survive very long, and the antigens targeted by the antibodies were unknown.

5.6   Hybridoma Technology: Monoclonal Antibodies of Known Specificity

To generate a cell producing an antibody of known specificity, Köhler and Milstein decided to fuse a normal B cell from the spleen of an immunized mouse with a myeloma cell line hoping to create an immortalized cell line producing monospecific antibodies. Köhler used a HAT cell culture medium (see below) that had previously been used by other research groups for the fusion of tumor cells. As previously used by Cotton, he also added Sendai virus to promote cell fusion. Sheep red blood cells (SRBC) were used as the antigen because they were known to induce a vigorous immune response and antibodies against SRBC could easily be detected with a plaque assay. In January 1975, after an initial failure due to contamination, Köhler observed clear green halos where the red blood cells had been destroyed. This was his "Eureka" moment, and he was overjoyed. The results were reproducible, and the seminal paper of Köhler and Milstein was accepted by Nature in May 1975. The method was then modified somewhat by Giovanni Galfré, a postdoctoral student, who substituted polyethylene glycol (PEG) instead of inactivated Sendai virus for cell fusion.

This groundbreaking technique paved the way for the facile production of identical monoclonal antibodies. It was now possible to produce homogeneous antibody preparations for diagnostics and the therapy of cancer and other illnesses. Antibodies produced with this technology against cell surface proteins have been especially useful in tracing cell development and differentiation and for analyzing cellular functions, thus playing a major role in the rapid development of the biological sciences. For their discovery of this method, Georges Köhler and César Milstein received the 1984 Nobel Prize in Physiology or Medicine, sharing it with Nils Jerne for his contributions to theories about the nature and control of the immune system (see Chap. 3).

5.7   Hybridoma Selection

As described above, hybridoma cells are produced by the fusion of B lymphocytes from the spleen of immunized mice with immortalizing myeloma cells. The antibody expressed by the B lymphocyte can be produced in relatively large quantities, since the myeloma cells are derived from antibody-producing plasma cells. To propagate the antibody-producing clones, it is only necessary to select against the unfused myeloma cells since the unfused spleen cells soon die. The selection is achieved using a HAT medium comprising *h*ypoxanthine, *a*minopterin, and *t*hymidine. Aminopterin, a folic acid antagonist, blocks an important synthetic route for producing purines and ultimately DNA and RNA. The hybrid cells contain the enzyme hypoxanthine-guanine phosphoribosyltransferase (HGPRT), which enables the production of the nucleotides via a second synthesis pathway (salvage pathway). Thymidine is also added since aminopterin blocks its synthesis. Myeloma cells do not contain HGPRT and soon die (see Fig. 5.1).

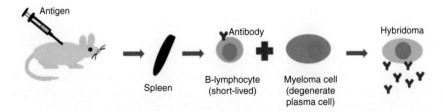

Fig. 5.1 Production of mouse monoclonal antibodies (mAbs). The spleen is a rich source of B lymphocytes, each of which expresses a unique antibody. The fusion of a B lymphocyte with a myeloma cell creates an immortalized hybridoma cell producing large amounts of identical mAbs

Monoclonal antibodies are usually made using the spleen cells from mice and rats because they are easy to handle. For ethical reasons, it is not possible to use the spleen cells of immunized humans. They are also difficult to handle, and the cultivation of human hybridoma cells has not been very successful.

5.8   First Approved Therapeutic Antibody

Muromonab-CD3 (trade name Orthoclone OKT3) was the first monoclonal antibody used for clinical applications (1986 for the prevention of tissue rejection after organ transplants). The development of other monoclonal antibodies for the treatment of various diseases was not very successful. This was partly because the foreign murine antibodies triggered an immune response; their interaction with human immune cells was also less effective than with murine immune cells. It was only after antibodies were produced containing a significant proportion of human sequences that further progress was made in developing therapeutic antibodies.

5.9   Humanization of Monoclonal Antibodies

In order not to impair the binding sites of the murine antibodies, initially only the constant domains of the antibodies were replaced by corresponding human sequences, resulting in the generation of so-called chimeric antibodies (Fig. 5.2). The use of the first chimeric antibody Rituxan/MabThera for the treatment of non-Hodgkin lymphoma was very successful. It was followed by the development of chimeric antibodies against several other cancers.

In order to further reduce the risk of a strong immune reaction, the parts of the variable regions not involved in antigen binding were replaced by human sequences. Only the murine CDRs (complementarity-determining regions) remained. These six regions, three per heavy and three per light chain, largely determine the binding affinity to the antigen due to their complementary structure. However, since the

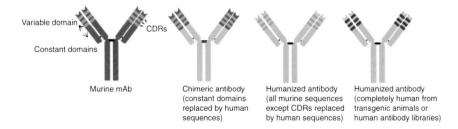

Fig. 5.2 Humanization of murine antibodies. The risk of a strong immune reaction against therapeutic antibodies has been significantly reduced by replacing the murine constant domains or all of the sequences except the CDRs, which largely determine the antibody specificity and affinity, with human sequences. To reduce the risk still further, completely human antibodies have been generated in transgenic animals or have been selected from large human antibody libraries

"humanized" antibodies often bound the antigen less strongly than the original murine antibody, small corrections usually had to be made in the sequences adjacent to the CDRs.

5.10   Human Antibodies from Transgenic Animals

To produce completely human antibodies and avoid the humanization procedure, a large part of the DNA coding for murine antibody genes was gradually replaced by the corresponding human DNA. These huge endeavors over many years finally resulted in the creation of transgenic mice producing human antibodies with very good binding properties after immunization with an antigen.

5.11   Human Antibody Libraries

To obtain human antibodies without the need for immunizing animals, the principles of in vivo antibody production and selection have been mimicked in vitro. This was achieved by isolating the genes coding for antibody heavy and light chains from a large number of B lymphocytes. Very large antibody libraries were then generated by randomly combining the heavy chain DNAs with the light chain DNAs. In an alternative method, large synthetic antibody libraries were created in vitro by introducing randomized amino acid sequences into the CDR regions of a particular human antibody scaffold chosen for its optimal properties regarding stability, production, and effector functions. With both methods it is possible to produce libraries comprising more than a billion different antibodies.

5.12   Selection of a Specific Antibody Using Phage Display

In vivo, the maturation and proliferation of a specific B cell are driven by the binding of an antigen (clonal selection). To mimic this selection process, the genes of an scFv (single-chain Fv; see Chap. 8) antibody library were fused to the bacteriophage gene coding for the five p3 proteins at the end of the phage particle used for docking onto the F pilus of *E. coli* bacteria. The p3-scFv fusion proteins can both bind antigens and dock onto *E. coli* to initiate infection. To select a particular antibody, the phage display library is incubated with an immobilized antigen on plastic microtiter plates (Fig. 5.3). Binding phage stick to the antigen, while the nonbinding phage are washed away. The binding phage are then eluted from the plate under conditions known to weaken the binding of the antibody to antigen such as low or high pH. To increase the number of binding phage for ease of handling, the eluted clones are allowed to proliferate by incubating them with *E. coli*. After harvesting, the proliferated phage from the *E.coli* medium are incubated once again with the immobilized antigen to decrease the number of any unspecific clones. This

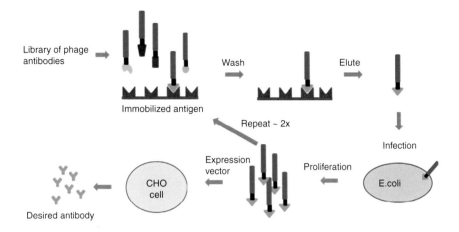

Fig. 5.3 Selection of specific antibodies using phage display. The antibody variable genes of a phage library displaying single-chain antibodies (scFvs) are fused with a bacteriophage gene coding for the p3 protein used for docking onto bacteria. The p3-scFv fusion protein enables the bacteriophage to bind antigens and infect *E. coli*. To select a specific scFv, the phage library is incubated with immobilized antigen on plastic microtiter plates followed by a wash step to remove non-binding phage. The remaining phage are eluted and multiplied by infecting *E. coli*. The phages are then subjected to additional cycles of antigen binding and elution to enrich for high-affinity antibodies. In a last step, the antibody genes in the DNA of the selected bacteriophages are inserted into an expression vector containing genes coding for the antibody constant domains, which is then transfected into CHO (Chinese hamster ovary) cells for production of full-length antibodies

procedure can be repeated a few times until the binding phage are sufficiently enriched with clones of the desired specificity. The antibody variable genes in the DNA of the selected phages are then cloned into an expression vector containing DNA coding for the antibody constant domains, which is then transfected into appropriate cells, such as the widely used CHO (Chinese hamster ovary) cells for production of full-length antibodies.

5.13   Production of Therapeutic Antibodies

The most common mammalian cell used for the production of antibodies is an immortalized cell line from the Chinese hamster ovary (CHO cell). Approximately 70% of all therapeutic proteins are produced in CHO cells after transfecting them with an expression vector containing genes coding for the proteins that are to be produced. Antibody titers of 5–10 g/L can be achieved in special fermenters. A high yield is especially important to reduce the costs of therapeutic antibodies, which are usually administered in relatively high quantities for treating cancer patients. For example, 3 g of the antibody Rituxan/MabThera (Rituximab) are needed pro patient for treating non-Hodgkin lymphoma.

5.14   GMP Conditions (Good Manufacturing Practice)

The manufacture of pharmaceuticals in the EU and United States is strictly regulated, in the EU by EudraLex (European Drug Regulatory Legislation) and in the United States by the Center for Drug Evaluation and Research (CDER, see the Federal Drug Agency (FDA) website). Precise guidelines on quality assurance, production, equipment, media, and clean room environment are specified. The manufacture of the antibody must be validated by a precise and detailed documentation of the reproducibility of the whole process and the results. The personnel must be qualified for working under GMP conditions. The quality of the air, the air pressure, the temperature, the sterilization of the devices, etc. must be constantly monitored. All cleaning steps must be carried out under GMP conditions, and the number of viral contaminants must be reduced to a minimum. As a rule, pharmaceutical companies try to comply with both the EU and US guidelines so that they can test their products and obtain market approval for administration to patients on both continents. Because of the high manufacturing costs, only larger companies are usually able to produce their own products under GMP conditions. Smaller and medium-sized companies contract the services of professional manufacturing companies.

Selected Literature

Almagro JC, Pedraza-Escalona M, Arrieta HI, Pérez-Tapia SM. Phage display libraries for antibody therapeutic discovery and development. Antibodies. 2019;8:44. https://doi.org/10.3390/antib8030044.

Chen WC, Murawsky CM. Strategies for generating diverse antibody repertoires using transgenic animals expressing human antibodies. Front Immunol. 2018;9:460. https://doi.org/10.3389/fimmu.2018.00460.

EU guidelines for good manufacturing practice for medicinal products for human and veterinary use. EudraLex Volume 4. https://ec.europa.eu/health/documents/eudralex/vol-4_en.

Joyce C, Burton DR, Briney B. Comparisons of the antibody repertoires of a humanized rodent and humans by high throughput sequencing. Sci Rep. 2020;10:1120. https://doi.org/10.1038/s41598-020-57764-7.

Köhler G, Milstein C. Continuous cultures of fused cells secreting antibody of predefined specificity. Nature. 1975;256:495–7.

Lee EC, Liang Q, Ali H, Bayliss L, Beasley A, Bloomfield-Gerdes T, et al. Complete humanization of the mouse immunoglobulin loci enables efficient therapeutic antibody discovery. Nat Biotechnol. 2014;32(4):356–63. https://doi.org/10.1038/nbt.2825.

Lerner R. Combinatorial antibody libraries: new advances, new immunological insights. Nat Rev Immunol. 2016;16:498–508. https://doi.org/10.1038/nri.2016.67.

Little M, editor. Recombinant antibodies for immunotherapy. 1st ed. Cambridge: Cambridge University Press; 2009.

Marks L. A healthcare revolution in the making—the story of César Milstein and monoclonal antibodies. What is biotechnology—special exhibition. 2013. https://www.whatisbiotechnology.org/index.php/exhibitions/milstein.

Parola C, Neumeier D, Reddy ST. Integrating high-throughput screening and sequencing for monoclonal antibody discovery and engineering. Immunology. 2018;153(1):31–41. https://doi.org/10.1111/imm.12838.

Pasello M, Mallano A, Flego M, et al. Construction of human naïve antibody gene libraries. Methods Mol Biol. 2018;1827:73–91. https://doi.org/10.1007/978-1-4939-8648-4_4.

Sinkovics JG. Discovery of the hybridoma principle in 1968-69 immortalization of the specific antibody-producing cell by fusion with a lymphoma cell. J Med. 1985;16(5–6):509–24.

US FDA current good manufacturing practice (CGMP) regulations. https://www.fda.gov/drugs/pharmaceutical-quality-resources/current-good-manufacturing-practice-cgmp-regulations.

Mediation of Tumor Cell Death by Naked Antibodies

Abstract

Most of the early monoclonal antibodies against target molecules on tumor cells for cancer therapy were naked antibodies without payloads. They can induce tumor cell death by the Fc-mediated effector functions of ADCC (antibody-dependent cellular cytotoxicity), ADCP (antibody-dependent cellular phagocytosis), and CDC (complement-dependent cytotoxicity) or by inhibiting the signaling pathway of growth hormone receptors on the tumor cell surface. The IgG1 subtype is usually chosen for eliminating tumor cells by ADCC and ADCP since it has a high affinity for the Fcγ receptors and is a potent activator of natural killer (NK) cells. Another approach has been to block the growth signals of angiogenesis (blood vessel formation) necessary for tumor nourishment. More recently, the use of antibodies directed against immune checkpoints on immune cells has made a major impact on the treatment of solid tumors. They have opened a window for treating cancers such as malignant melanomas that were previously resistant to therapy. Tumors that are particularly amenable to treatment with IC inhibitors are characterized by a high mutation rate and a significant number of tumor-infiltrating lymphocytes (TILs). However, not all patients with these so-called "hot" tumors respond due to the highly immunosuppressive tumor microenvironment. Recent advances in our understanding of these resistance mechanisms could provide new strategies for combining antibodies directed at ICs with other complementary therapeutic approaches.

6.1 Introduction

The first therapeutic antibody to be approved for treating cancer was the murine monoclonal antibody Panorex (Edrecolomab) in 1995. It is directed against the 17-1A antigen on carcinomas and was used to treat colorectal cancer. However, the

M. Little, *Antibodies for Treating Cancer*,
https://doi.org/10.1007/978-3-030-72599-0_6

real breakthrough in the field came 3 years later with the approval of the chimeric antibody Rituxan/MabThera (rituximab) in 1997 for the treatment of non-Hodgkin lymphoma (NHL) and the humanized antibody Herceptin (trastuzumab) in 1998 for the treatment of breast cancer. These were followed by an increasing number of therapeutic antibodies that were either humanized or completely human.

6.2   Antibodies Targeting Antigens on Tumor Cells

Death Signals: Apoptosis

The binding of an antibody to some antigens on the cell surface can trigger signals for programmed cell death (apoptosis, Fig. 6.1a). The strongest apoptotic signals arise when the antibody binds a member of the tumor necrosis factor (TNF) receptor family for ligands such as TNF-related apoptosis-inducing ligand (TRAIL), Fas, and TNF-α. Binding of these ligands to their cognate receptors induces receptor aggregation and the formation of a macromolecular complex, coined DISC

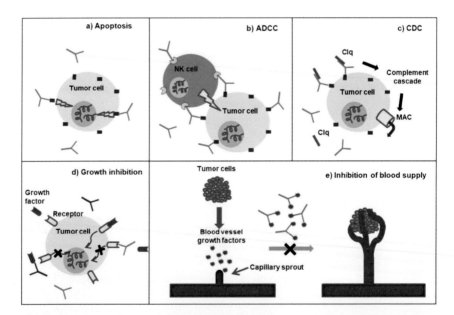

Fig. 6.1 Mechanisms of cancer therapy with naked mAbs. The antibodies bind either to tumor-associated antigens (TAAs) or to growth factors/growth factor receptors; (**a**) binding to some cell surface proteins induces programmed cell death by the proteolytic caspase cascade (apoptosis); (**b**) binding of the antibody Fc domain to receptors on NK (natural killer) activates ADCC (antibody-dependent cellular cytotoxicity); (**c**) binding of the antibody Fc domain to C1q, the first component of the complement cascade, initiates CDC (complement-dependent cytotoxicity) with the formation of the membrane attack complex (MAC); (**d**) blockage of growth factors or their receptors; (**e**) blockage of blood vessel growth factors or their receptors

(death-inducing signaling complex), which promotes the activation of the proteolytic caspase cascade leading to apoptosis. However, the outcome of clinical trials with monoclonal antibody agonists against TRAIL receptors has been disappointing. Antibodies binding to other receptors or cell surface proteins can also induce apoptotic signals, but these are usually not sufficient to destroy the cell. They can however complement other mechanisms of action described below.

Fc-Mediated Effector Functions

ADCC (antibody-dependent cellular cytotoxicity, Fig. 6.1b), CDC (complement-dependent cytotoxicity, Fig. 6.1c), and ADCP (antibody-dependent cellular phagocytosis) have already been described in Chap. 2. The IgG1 and IgG3 subtypes have the highest binding affinities to the Fcγ receptors. However, the IgG3 subtype is not usually chosen as a therapeutic format due to its long hinge region and polymorphic nature, which are thought to increase the risk of proteolysis and immunogenicity. IgG2 and IgG4 have only weak effector functions; IgG4 is usually chosen as the most suitable format for those antibodies where only the binding function without Fc effector functions is required such as for blocking immune checkpoints (see below).

Optimal induction of ADCC is dependent on the abundance of the target molecule on tumor cells, for which the minimal requirement per cell is about 10^5 to 10^6 molecules. Cells with target densities less than 10^5 per cell are less likely to induce ADCC and will not be damaged. The best tumor-associated antigens (TAAs) are therefore those that are significantly overexpressed on tumor cells and only expressed at low levels on normal tissues.

6.3   Activating Fcγ Receptors

The most relevant activating FcγRs for therapeutic antibodies are FcγRIIA (CD32A, on monocytes, macrophages, neutrophils, and dendritic cells) and FcγRIIIA (CD16A, on natural killer (NK) cells, monocytes, and macrophages). However, the clinical efficacy of antibodies mediating ADCC appears to be mainly dependent on the activation of NK cells through the FcRIIIA receptor. Both of the activating FcγRs have two allelic variants: FcγRIIA-H131/R131 with the H131 allele having an overall higher affinity for Fc than the R131 allele and FcγRIIIA-V158/F158 with the V158 allele having a higher affinity for Fc than the F158 allele. Lymphoma patients expressing the higher-affinity FcγRIIIA-V158 were reported to have improved clinical outcomes when treated with anti-CD20 and anti-HER2 antibodies (see below) compared to patients homozygous for the lower-affinity FcγRIIIA-F158. This finding stimulated extensive efforts to engineer Fc domains with improved binding for the V158 allele.

Enhancement of Fc Effector Functions

Mutations have been introduced into the Fc domain that enhance ADCC and ADCP by increasing its affinity for both of the FcRIIA and FcRIIIA receptors. Alternatively, the activation of tumor cell killing by NK cells can be increased by removing fucose from the glycan at position 297. The fucose molecule is close to the FcγR binding site and appears to sterically impair binding between the antibody and Fc receptor. Cell lines that do not synthesize fucose molecules have therefore been developed for the production of therapeutic antibodies. Defucosylated antibodies were shown to have up to 50-fold enhanced affinity for FcγRIIIA. Other mutations have been introduced to increase binding to complement. To increase the half-life of therapeutic antibodies, mutations have been introduced that increase binding to the neonatal receptor FcRn at pH 6.0.

Rituxan/MabThera for Treating Non-Hodgkin's Lymphoma (NHL)

ADCC and CDC are the major mechanisms of tumor cell depletion employed by the chimeric antibody Rituxan/MabThera (rituximab), which was the first antibody for cancer therapy comprising a significant portion of human sequences. It was genetically engineered by replacing the constant domains of a murine antibody with corresponding human sequences. In 1997, it was approved in the United States for use in relapsed/refractory indolent non-Hodgkin lymphoma (NHL) and subsequently for other B-cell malignancies.

Non-Hodgkin lymphoma (NHL) is a malignant disease that affects the lymphatic system and is the fifth most common cancer after breast, prostate, lung, and colon cancers. Malignant lymphomas are subdivided into non-Hodgkin lymphoma (NHL) and Hodgkin lymphoma, whereby the NHL family of cancers are quite diverse. Malignant lymphocytes can settle anywhere in the body, for example, in the lymph nodes, spleen, bone marrow, blood, and other organs where they form a lymphoma, which is the most common form of blood cancer. About 80% of all NHL are derived from B lymphocytes and about 20% from T lymphocytes. The diffuse large B cell lymphomas and the indolent (slow growing) follicular lymphomas are the most common.

Rituxan binds with high affinity to the CD20 antigen, a glycosylated transmembrane protein expressed on the surface of normal and malignant B lymphocytes but not on normal tissues. It is also not expressed on B-cell progenitors or mature plasma cells so that B lymphocytes can be regenerated after therapy; recovery to normal levels takes about 6–12 months. It has demonstrated an impressive efficacy and safety profile both as monotherapy in first-line treatment (induction therapy) and maintenance of progression-free survival (PFS), and in combination with chemotherapy for the treatment of patients with various CD20-expressing malignancies such as chronic lymphocytic leukemia (CLL), the most common form of leukemia in adults.

Rituxan also appears to sensitize chemoresistant cells to chemotherapeutic drugs. In an initial study in patients with low-grade NHL ($n = 35$), Rituxan combined with cyclophosphamide, doxorubicin, vincristine, and prednisone (CHOP) resulted in an overall response rate of 100%, whereby 63% of the patients had a complete response with no significant increase in toxicity. The benefits of immuno/chemotherapy were also clearly demonstrated in the first randomized study comparing MabThera-CHOP (M-CHOP) with a standard CHOP regimen in 399 previously untreated elderly patients with diffuse large B-cell lymphoma (DLBCL). The study (LNH-98.5) was carried out by the Groupe d'Etudes des Lymphomes de l'Adulte (GELA). Seventy-six percent of patients treated with M-CHOP showed complete responses compared to 63% of patients treated only with CHOP. After 2 years the overall survival (OS) was 70% for M-CHOP versus 57% for CHOP alone, and after 10 years the overall survival was 43.5% for M-CHOP compared with 27.6% for CHOP alone.

In the prescribing information, it is recommended to administer the first dose of Rituxan as an intravenous infusion at 50 mg/h. The rate is increased by 50 mg/h every 30 min until a maximum infusion rate is achieved of 400 mg/h; treatment is terminated after reaching a total dose of 375 mg/m^2. Although Rituxan proved to be particularly well tolerated by patients, the safety information includes a boxed warning for fatal infusion-related reactions. Deaths have occurred within 24 h of infusion.

6.4   Growth Inhibition of Tumor Cells

Growth factor receptors on the cell surface are activated by the binding of soluble growth factor ligands. One of the best characterized receptors is EGFR (epidermal growth factor receptor) that is expressed by nearly all adult tissues with the exception of hematopoietic cells. It is overexpressed by many tumors and is correlated with a poor prognosis. The activated signaling pathway stimulates cell proliferation, migration, and invasion correlating with disease progression, reduced survival, and resistance to chemotherapy. Blocking the signaling pathway by antibodies inhibits the growth of cancer cells (Fig. 6.1d).

Herceptin for Treating Breast Cancer

Herceptin (trastuzumab) is a humanized IgG1 antibody against HER2, a tyrosine kinase receptor that is overexpressed in many cancers but primarily in ovarian and breast carcinomas. HER2 is distinct from EGFR (see below) in that it has no known ligand and functions by dimerizing with itself or heterodimerizing with other growth factor receptors to enhance their activation. Herceptin functions by preventing ligand-independent HER2 signaling and by inducing ADCC, which probably explains why cancer cells with particularly high expressions of HER2 are more susceptible to therapy. The HER2 gene (also known as HER2/neu and ErbB2 gene) is amplified in 20–30% of early-stage breast cancers where it can be expressed up to 100 times more than in normal cells. These cancers have the second poorest prognosis among the cancer breast subtypes.

The prescribing information for treating metastatic breast cancer recommends an initial dosing load of 4 mg/kg infused over 90 min and subsequent weekly doses of 2 mg/kg infused over 30 min to be given until disease progression. Although Herceptin has a high affinity for HER2 and can be administered in relatively high doses because of its low toxicity, approximately 70% of HER2+ patients do not respond to treatment and nearly all patients develop a resistance to treatment. A small percentage of patients develop a serious cardiac dysfunction. Nevertheless, Herceptin remains an important part of the treatment regime for HER2+ tumors, particularly with the aim of eliminating micrometastases at an early stage.

The combination of Herceptin with chemotherapy has been shown to increase both survival and response rate, in comparison to trastuzumab alone. In 2012, Lorenzo Mojo and colleagues in Milan published an analysis of eight studies comparing the efficacy and safety of Herceptin alone, or in combination with chemotherapy, or no treatment, or standard chemotherapy alone, in 11,991 women with HER2-positive early breast cancer including women with locally advanced breast cancer. They concluded that if 1000 women were given standard chemotherapy alone (with no Herceptin), then about 900 would survive and 5 would have experienced heart toxicities. If 1000 women were treated with standard chemotherapy and Herceptin for 1 year, about 933 would survive and 26 would have serious heart toxicity. Furthermore, about 740 women would have no recurrence of disease after treatment with Herceptin/chemotherapy, which is 95 more than for women who only receive chemotherapy.

Herceptin is now often used together with the humanized IgG1 antibody Perjeta (pertuzumab) that inhibits the heterodimerization of HER2 with the other HER receptors, HER1 and HER3. The available evidence suggests that they can act synergistically in the treatment of HER2+ breast cancers. The beneficial effects of a combination therapy were demonstrated in the large randomized "CLEOPATRA" study carried out with 808 patients who received either placebo plus trastuzumab plus docetaxel (control group) or pertuzumab plus trastuzumab plus docetaxel (pertuzumab group) as first-line treatment. The median progression-free survival was 12.4 months in the control group, as compared with 18.5 months in the pertuzumab group, with a favorable overall survival in an interim analysis and no increase in cardiac toxic effects.

Erbitux for Treating Colorectal Cancer

Erbitux (cetuximab) is a chimeric IgG1 antibody against the epidermal growth factor receptor (EGFR) for the treatment of colorectal cancer, one of the most frequent cancers (see Chap. 10). It induces apoptosis in tumor cells by blocking ligand binding and receptor dimerization. ADCC has also been implicated in its mechanism of action. Approximately 75% of patients with metastatic colorectal cancer have EGFR-expressing tumors, many of which have mutations in the Ras family of proteins comprising HRAS, KRAS, and NRAS that constitutively activate the EGFR signaling pathway.

Approximately 60% of metastatic colorectal tumors have the wild-type KRAS. However, only 35–40% of patients with wild-type KRAS benefit from anti-EGFR treatment. Originally approved by the FDA in 2004, Erbitux was restricted in 2009 to the treatment of metastatic colorectal cancer tumors expressing wild-type KRAS (United States and Canada) or the wild-type RAS (EU and elsewhere). This decision was based on a clinical trial by Christos Karapetis and colleagues in 2008 to investigate the benefits of Erbitux for patients with colorectal cancer who have not responded to chemotherapy. The same decision was made for the use of the completely human IgG2 antibody Vectibix (panitumumab) after it was shown that no benefits were obtained for patients with NRAS mutations.

In the 2008 trial, Erbitux was applied intravenously to one group of patients with a dose of 400 mg/m^2 over 2 h on day 1 followed by an infusion of 250 mg/m^2 over 1 h, once a week until the disease progressed or until the toxic effects could no longer be tolerated. This group also received best supportive care. The second group only received best supportive care. For patients with wild-type KRAS tumors, treatment with Erbitux as compared to supportive care alone significantly improved overall survival (median, 9.5 versus 4.8 months and progression-free survival 3.7 months versus 1.9 months). Among patients with mutated KRAS tumors, there was no significant difference between those who were treated with Erbitux and those who received supportive care alone with respect to overall survival.

However, the results of a recent multicenter, open-label, randomized, controlled, phase III trial coordinated by the Cancer Research UK Southampton Clinical Trials Unit in patients with wild-type KRAS resectable colorectal liver metastasis (the New EPOC trial) showed a significant disadvantage of Erbitux in terms of overall survival. Median progression-free survival was 22.2 months in the chemotherapy alone group and 15.5 months in the chemotherapy plus cetuximab group. However, the median overall survival was 81.0 months in the chemotherapy alone group and 55.4 months in the chemotherapy plus Erbitux group. The investigators warn that Erbitux should not be used in this setting. Furthermore, they point out that although studies using anti-EGFR in advanced disease were mostly positive, those in the adjuvant setting were not, with a trend towards detrimental outcomes in older patients. Since in the New EPOC study most patients were operable with a predominant effect likely to be on micrometastatic disease, this would be consistent with the adjuvant anti-EGFR therapy data.

The reason for the surprising outcome of the New EPOC trial is a matter of speculation. One interesting correlation is that a high expression of the microRNA miR-31–3p in primary colorectal cancer of patients with metastatic disease treated with Erbitux or Vectibix has been shown to be associated with resistance to anti-EGFR and disease progression. MicroRNAs (miRNA) are small non-coding RNA molecules that play a key role in the regulation of intracellular processes through post-transcriptional regulation of gene expression. Those controlling the expression of oncogenes and tumor suppressor genes are frequently deregulated in cancer cells.

Naked mAbs that have been approved for cancer therapy are shown in Table 6.1.

Table 6.1 Naked mAbs approved for cancer therapy

Brand name	INN	Format	Target	First approval	Indication of first approval[a]
Panorex	Edrecolomab	Murine IgG1	EpCAM	1995[b,c]	Colorectal cancer
Rituxan/ MabThera	Rituximab	Chimeric IgG1	CD20	1997	Non-Hodgkin lymphoma (NHL)
Herceptin	Trastuzumab	Humanized IgG1	HER2	1998	Breast cancer
Campath/ Lemtrada	Alemtuzumab	Humanized IgG1	CD52	2001	Chronic myeloid leukemia (CML)
Erbitux	Cetuximab	Chimeric IgG1	EGFR	2004	Colorectal cancer
Avastin	Bevacizumab	Humanized IgG1	VEGF-A	2004	Colorectal cancer
Vectibix	Panitumumab	Human IgG2	EGFR	2006	Colorectal cancer
Removab	Catumaxomab	Bispecific rat/ mouse hybrid IgG	CD3 and EpCAM	2009[c]	Malignant ascites
Arzerra	Ofatumumab	Human IgG1	CD20	2009	Chronic lymphocytic leukemia (CLL)
Yervoy	Ipilimumab	Human IgG1	CTLA-4	2011	Malignant melanoma
Perjeta	Pertuzumab	Humanized IgG1	HER2	2012	Breast cancer
Gazyva/ Gazyvaro	Obinutuzumab	Humanized glyco-engineered IgG1	CD20	2013	Chronic lymphocytic leukemia
Cyramza	Ramucirumab	Human IgG1	VEGFR2	2014	Gastric cancer
Blincyto	Blinatumomab	Murine bispecific tandem scFv	CD3 and CD19	2014	Acute lymphoblastic leukemia (ALL)
Opdivo	Nivolumab	Human IgG4	PD-1	2014	Melanoma, non-small cell lung cancer
Keytruda	Pembrolizumab	Human IgG4	PD-1	2014	Melanoma
Portrazza	Necitumumab	Human IgG1	EGFR	2015	Non-small cell lung cancer
Unituxin	Dinutuximab	Chimeric IgG1	GD2	2015	Neuroblastoma
Darzalex	Daratumumab	Human IgG1	CD38	2015	Multiple myeloma
Empliciti	Elotuzumab	Humanized IgG1	SLAMF7	2015	Multiple myeloma
Lartruvo	Olaratumab	Human IgG1	PDGFRα	2016	Soft tissue sarcoma
Tecentriq	Atezolizumab	Humanized IgG1	PD-L1	2016	Bladder cancer
Bavencio	Avelumab	Human IgG1	PD-L1	2017	Merkel cell carcinoma
Imfinzi	Durvalumab	Human IgG1	PD-L1	2017	Bladder cancer
Libtayo	Cemiplimab	Human IgG4	PD-1	2018	Cutaneous squamous cell carcinoma

Table 6.1   (continued)

Brand name	INN	Format	Target	First approval	Indication of first approval[a]
Sarclisa	Isatuximab	Chimeric IgG1	CD38	2020	Multiple myeloma
Monjuvi	Tafasitamab	Humanized IgG1 Fc engineered	CD19	2020	Diffuse large B-cell lymphoma

INN International nonproprietary name, *EpCAM* epithelial cell adhesion molecule, *CD antigen* cluster of differentiation antigen, *HER2* human epidermal growth factor receptor 2, *EGFR* epidermal growth factor receptor, *VEGF-A* vascular endothelial growth factor A, *VEGFR2* VEGF receptor 2, *CTLA-4* cytotoxic T-lymphocyte-associated antigen 4, *131I* conjugated with iodine-131, *90Y* conjugated with yttrium-90, *PD-1* programmed cell death protein 1, *PD-L1* PD-ligand 1, *GD2* ganglioside D2 antigen, *SLAMF7 (CD319)* signaling lymphocytic activation molecule family member 7, *PDGFRα* platelet-derived growth factor receptor alpha
[a]In the United States if not stated otherwise
[b]Only in Germany
[c]Voluntarily withdrawn from the market

A complete and current list of INNs for therapeutic antibodies approved or under regulatory review in the United States and EU can be found on the Antibody Society's website—http://www.antibodysociety.org/news/approved-antibodies/.

6.5   Antibodies Targeting Angiogenesis (Blood Vessel Formation)

When a group of cancer cells has reached a certain size, the tumor can no longer grow without nourishing blood vessels. Tumor cells then release special growth factors such as VEGF (vascular endothelial growth factor) which bind to receptors in the endothelium (the inner layer of cells in blood vessels) and cause budding. The concentration gradient of VEGF directs the growth of the capillary sprouts towards the tumor. Antibodies against angiogenic factors (see Fig. 6.1e) or their receptors inhibit tumor growth.

Avastin for Treating Solid Tumors

Avastin (bevacizumab) is a humanized IgG1 antibody against vascular endothelial growth factor A (VEGF-A) that inhibits angiogenesis. It was first approved in the United States in 2004 in combination with standard chemotherapy for treating metastatic colon cancer. It has since been approved for some lung cancers, renal cancers, ovarian cancers, and glioblastoma. In a study of 813 patients with previously untreated metastatic colorectal cancer by Herbert Hurwitz and colleagues published in 2004, about one half of the patients were randomly assigned to receive irinotecan, bolus fluorouracil, and leucovorin (IFL) plus bevacizumab (5 mg/kg of body weight every 2 weeks) and one half to receive IFL plus placebo. The median duration of survival was 20.3 months in the group given IFL plus bevacizumab, as compared with 15.6 months in the group given IFL plus placebo. The median duration of progression-free survival was 10.6 months in the group given IFL plus bevacizumab, as compared with 6.2 months in the group given IFL plus placebo. Common side effects included nose bleeds, headache, high blood pressure, and rash.

However, in a study of 2672 patients with stages II and III colon carcinoma published by Carmen Allegra and colleagues in 2011 for investigating the benefit of Avastin in combination with chemotherapy for adjuvant therapy (NSABP Protocol C-08), they found no significant disease-free survival (DFS). They concluded that the use of Avastin cannot be recommended for use in the adjuvant treatment of patients with colon cancer.

Cyramza for Treating Colorectal Cancer

Cyramza (ramucirumab) is a fully human IgG1 antibody that binds with high affinity to the extracellular domain of VEGFR2 and blocks the binding of the VEGFR ligands VEGF-A, VEGF-C, and VEGF-D. It was approved by the FDA in 2015 for the treatment of patients with metastatic colorectal cancer with disease progression on or after prior therapy with Avastin, oxaliplatin, and fluoropyrimidine. The approval was based on the results of the RAISE trial, a phase III study published by Josep Tabernero and colleagues in 2015 which compared Cyramza plus irinotecan, folinic acid, and 5-fluorouracil (FOLFIRI) to FOLFIRI alone. The median overall survival was 13.3 months for Cyramza plus chemotherapy versus 11.7 months for chemotherapy alone. The study group concluded that Cyramza plus FOLFIRI significantly improved overall survival as second-line treatment for patients with metastatic colorectal carcinoma. Cyramza has also been approved for use in the treatment of other solid tumors such as advanced gastric cancer, non-small cell lung cancer (NSCLC) and hepatocellular carcinoma (HCC). However, it failed to improve progression-free survival for metastatic breast cancer or to improve overall survival in liver cancer.

6.6   Activation of Immune Cells by Monoclonal Antibodies

Tumor-Infiltrating Lymphocytes

Solid tumors are often infiltrated with some or all of the white blood cells described in Chap. 2 in varying proportions depending on the tumor type and stage of disease. These tumor-infiltrating lymphocytes (TILs) were used by Steven Rosenberg and colleagues at the US National Cancer Institute in Bethesda, Maryland, to develop an adoptive T-cell transfer therapy for treating patients with melanoma. TILs from the resected tumors of patients with melanoma are expanded with a high dose of IL-2 for a few weeks and then further expanded by activating the CD3 receptor of the T lymphocytes with an anti-CD3 monoclonal antibody for about 2 weeks. The cells are then infused back into the patient. To improve the access of the TILs to the tumor, a chemotherapy regimen is preferably administered 1 week prior to the infusion. After infusion, the patients are infused with high-dose IL-2 or other cytokine support. A tumor reduction of 50% was found in about half of the patients, and in a clinical trial of 93 melanoma patients treated with TILs, 19 had complete remissions for over 3 years.

The potential of TILs for treating a large number of other solid tumors is now under investigation. They are also attractive targets for the development of activation strategies using monoclonal antibodies to break the immunosuppressive stranglehold imposed by the tumor microenvironment (see immune checkpoints and resistance mechanisms below).

Antibodies for Activating Costimulatory Receptors on T Cells

The activation of immune cells is tightly regulated by a large number of stimulatory and inhibitory receptors on the cell surface which bind to complementary ligands on the surface of antigen-presenting cells and non-immune cells such as tumor cells. Particularly cytotoxic T cells are very much in the focus of cancer immunotherapy because of their very potent killing capacity. As already described in Chap. 2, the mechanism of T-cell activation requires a second costimulatory signal in addition to the signal provided by the T-cell receptor. An overview of the costimulatory receptors on the surface of T cells and their complementary ligand on non-immune cells including tumor cells is shown in Fig. 6.2.

To enhance a T-cell response against tumor cells, agonistic monoclonal antibodies have been developed against various costimulatory receptors shown in Fig. 6.2. For example, agonist antibodies against CD40 stimulate antigen presentation by dendritic cells and mAbs to OX40 and 4-1BB activate T cells while reducing the activity of T regulatory cells (Tregs). However, as described in the following report on the administration of a costimulatory antibody to healthy human probands, there is always a risk of unleashing a potentially dangerous cytokine storm.

The TeGenero Bombshell

On March 13, 2006, six probands at Northwick Park Hospital in Harrow near London were infused with the antibody theralizumab (aka TGN1412), a humanized IgG4 monoclonal antibody against the costimulatory receptor CD28 on T cells developed by the German startup firm TeGenero. It was originally selected for clinical development because it acted as a "superagonist" able to activate T cells without a primary signal from the T-cell receptor. As it appeared to have a stimulatory mode of action on regulatory T cells, it was thought that the antibody may be effective for the treatment of multiple sclerosis and arthritis.

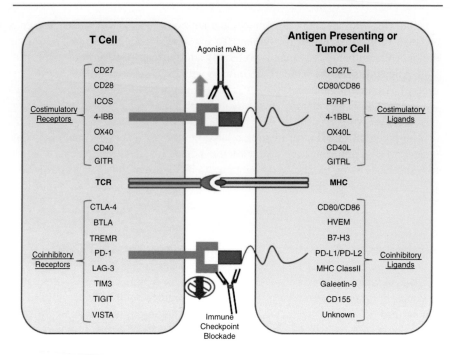

Fig. 6.2 Costimulatory receptors and immune checkpoints on T cells. The highly complex process of immune cell activation and regulation involves a diverse array of costimulatory and inhibitory signals for maintaining self-tolerance and modulating immune responses. (From Zahavi D and Weiner L. Antibodies 2020, 9, 34. https://doi.org/10.3390/antib9030034. Permission for use according to creative commons license (http://creativecommons.org/licenses/by/4.0/))

The infusions took place with only 10-min intervals between each patient and were administered at a dose of 0.1 mg/kg for 3–6 min. Shortly after the last injection, the first patient to be treated, David Oakley, complained of an unbearable headache. The 34-year-old also suffered from palpitations and severe pains in the kidneys and lungs. He also vomited large quantities of bile and had to fight for his life during the next few days in the intensive care unit. The other probands fared no better; they were also vomiting and experiencing severe pain. Between 12 and 16 h postdose, they became critically ill, with pulmonary infiltrates and lung injury, renal failure, and disseminated intravascular coagulation. Some of them felt that they were freezing, and the head and limbs of one proband were so swollen that the press called him the "Elephant Man." Prolonged cardiovascular shock and acute respiratory distress syndrome developed in two patients, who required intensive organ support for 8 and 16 days. Fortunately, all six volunteers survived, although their long-term prognosis is unknown. The 20-year-old proband Ryan Wilson later had to have all of his toes and the tips of several fingers amputated.

The young men who received £2000 for participating in the study were all victims of a cytokine storm released by immune cells after the inordinate activation of the T cells. They still suffer from long-term effects such as memory loss and fatigue.

Initially, they received only minimal compensation for their ordeal since TeGenero went bankrupt shortly afterwards, and the US company Parexel, which carried out the study, was unwilling to accept responsibility. However, after UK law firms started preparing the initiation of legal proceedings against Parexel's insurers, the two sides got together and agreed upon the payment of substantial compensations.

The fairly high starting dose for TGN1412 was based on animal experiments in which doses as high as 500 times those used in the clinical trial showed no significant side effects. One of the possible reasons was revealed a few years later when it was found that the CD4+ effector memory T cells of *Macaca fascicularis*, the primate used for preclinical safety testing, did not express CD28. It seems doubtful, however, whether this finding alone could explain the lack of an immediate immune response in monkeys as seen in the human probands.

Even when all the mitigating circumstances are considered, the fact remains that an antibody known to have a superagonist effect on activating T cells was administered at relatively high doses without any significant intervals between each proband. The highly publicized effects of TGN 1412 on the six healthy young men sent shockwaves through the companies developing therapeutic antibodies and the international regulatory authorities responsible for approving clinical trials. New guidelines were drawn up raising the standards of safety to a level where another catastrophe similar to that caused by TGN 1412 would be highly unlikely, if not impossible (see Chap. 10).

6.7   Antibodies Targeting Immune Checkpoints (ICs) on T Cells

James Allison and Tasuku Honjo received the Nobel Prize in Physiology or Medicine in 2018 after showing that CTLA-4 (cytotoxic T-lymphocyte-associated protein 4) and PD-1 (programmed cell death protein 1) were immune checkpoints that inhibited the activation of immune cells. On blocking the activation of these checkpoints with antibodies, they were able to show an antitumor effect of the immune cells. The inhibitory receptors on immune cells are essential for maintaining self-tolerance and regulating the immune response in order to prevent an overshooting immune reaction with collateral tissue damage. Their importance as a basis for an IC-based immunotherapy highlighted the importance of tumor immunology and opened a window on potential new therapeutic approaches. An overview of the immune checkpoint inhibitors on T cells and their corresponding ligands on normal non-immune cells and tumor cells is shown in Fig. 6.2.

The CD28 family of receptors on T cells is a subgroup of the immunoglobulin superfamily that plays a particularly prominent role in the positive and negative regulation of T-cell function. Two family members, CD28 and ICOS (inducible T-cell costimulator), act as positive regulators of T-cell function, while another three, BTLA (B- and T-lymphocyte attenuator), CTLA-4, and PD-1, act as inhibitory ICs. The ligands for the CD28 receptor family include the equally prominent B7 family of proteins: B7.1 (CD80), B7.2 (CD86), ICOS-L, PD-L1, PD-L2, B7-H3, and B7-H4.

Yervoy (ipilimumab) was the first antibody against an IC to be approved for cancer therapy in 2011 for treating melanoma and in 2018 for treating renal cell carcinoma. It is a human IgG1 antibody directed against the IC CTLA-4, which is constitutively expressed on Treg cells and transiently expressed at the cell-cell interaction boundary on other T-cell subsets, especially CD4+ T cells, upon activation. Before activation it is mainly located in intracellular vesicles. After being expressed at the immunological synapse, it binds to two ligands of the B7 family, CD80 and CD86, with a much higher affinity than CD28, thus outcompeting it and preventing the transmission of a costimulatory signal. Figure 6.3 shows an example of the inhibition of helper T cells after activation by a dendritic cell in the draining lymph node of a tumor. CTLA-4 on Tregs is also able to deplete CD80 and CD86 from the surface of antigen-presenting cells by a process of trans-endocytosis, which plays an important role in mediating the immune suppression of bystander cells by reducing the availability of these stimulatory proteins to CD28. Yervoy is thus thought to exert its T-cell-activating effect by depleting the population of Tregs by ADCC/ADCP and inhibiting the action of CD28 on activated T cells. Importantly, Yervoy is an IgG1 antibody with strong effector functions for ADCC/ADCP. Another anti-CTLA-4 antibody that has been developed for cancer therapy, tremelimumab, is an IgG2 antibody with a much weaker potential for mediating ADCC/ADCP, which may partly explain its failure in late-stage clinical trials.

Keytruda (pembrolizumab, humanized IgG4), *Opdivo* (nivolumab, human IgG4), and *Libtayo* (cemiplimab, human IgG4) are directed against the immune checkpoint inhibitor PD-1. *Tecentriq* (atezolizumab, humanized IgG1), *Bavencio*

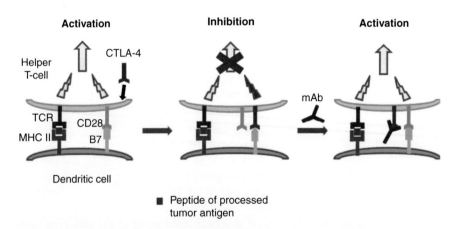

Fig. 6.3 Inhibition of helper T-cell activation by CTLA-4. After activation of CD4+ helper T cells by dendritic cells presenting tumor antigen peptides in a draining lymph node, intracellular CTLA-4 is transported to the cell surface where it outcompetes the B7 ligands, CD80, and CD86, for binding to the activating receptor CD28. The blockade of T-cell activation is inhibited by a therapeutic antibody against CTLA-4. Another major inhibitory mechanism of the IgG1 mAb Yervoy is ascribed to the depletion of Tregs, which constitutively express CTLA-4 on the cell surface, by ADCC/ADCP

(avelumab, human IgG1), and *Imfinzi* (durvalumab, human IgG1) are directed against PD-L1, a complementary ligand of PD-1 on various other cells including antigen-presenting cells and tumor cells. PD-1 is a major checkpoint inhibitor with a kinase function that is switched on after engagement with its ligand during T-cell activation by an antigen-presenting cell or by a tumor cell. Its kinase activity initiates a signaling pathway that interferes with the signaling pathways initiated by activation of the T-cell receptor and the costimulatory receptor CD28. It thus provides an important negative feedback mechanism to prevent an overshooting T-cell reaction.

Keytruda and Opdivo were originally approved for the treatment of melanoma in 2014. Since then, they and other antibodies directed against PD-1 or its ligand have been approved for the treatment of a variety of other solid tumors including bladder cancer, non-small cell lung cancer, liver cancer, gastric cancer, triple-negative breast cancer, urothelial carcinoma, Merkel cell carcinoma, cutaneous squamous cell carcinoma, small cell lung cancer, and renal cancer.

Successful Combination Therapy of Opdivo and Yervoy

Opdivo and Yervoy are directed against checkpoint inhibitors employing different mechanisms of inhibitory action. It was therefore surmised that a combination of the two antibodies might result in a much more effective therapeutic response than single antibody therapy. The results of a 5-year follow-up of a phase III clinical trial (CheckMate 067) to assess the benefits of combining Yervoy with Opdivo were published in October 2019. The trial randomly assigned 945 patients with previously untreated advanced melanoma into three groups that received one of the following regimens: Opdivo (1 mg/kg) plus Yervoy (3 mg/kg) every 3 weeks for four doses followed by Opdivo (3 mg/kg every 2 weeks); Opdivo (3 mg/kg every 2 weeks) plus Yervoy-matched placebo; or Yervoy (3 mg/kg every 3 weeks for four doses) plus Opdivo-matched placebo.

After a minimum follow-up period of 5 years, the median overall survival was more than 60 months in the Opdivo plus Yervoy group and 36.9 months in the Opdivo group compared to 19.9 months in the Yervoy group. Overall survival after 5 years was 52% Opdivo plus Yervoy, 44% Opdivo, and 26% Yervoy. Grade 3 or 4 treatment-related adverse events occurred in 59% (Opdivo plus Yervoy), 23% (Opdivo), and 28% (Yervoy) of the patients. The most common adverse events were diarrhea, colon inflammation, and high levels of lipase.

Antibodies directed against CTLA-4 and PD-1/PD-L1 are now being used as first-line treatments for cancer therapy. Their success has spurred investigations into the application of antibodies against the other immune checkpoints shown in Fig. 6.2 for cancer therapy. Many opportunities remain for exploring the best combinations of these antibodies with one another or with antibodies directed against other targets affecting tumor cell proliferation or immunosuppression (see resistance mechanisms below). Other immune cells are controlled by checkpoints that could also be exploited for cancer therapy. NK cells, for example, are potent cytotoxic cells regulated by a large number of stimulatory and inhibitory receptors such as KIR (killer inhibitory receptor). Antibodies against these potential targets could possibly be combined with the IC antibodies mentioned above to augment the destruction of tumor cells.

6.8   Mechanisms of Resistance

Immunoediting

Tumor cells evolve a variety of mechanisms to avoid immune recognition. It has been postulated that an accumulation of random critical mutations eventually gives rise to clones that are able to evade the immune system, a process known as immunoediting. Mechanisms of escape from immune surveillance include downregulation of tumor antigens or the antigen-presenting MHC class I complex and induction of alternative growth signaling pathways. Tumor cells have also escaped destruction by upregulating the expression of ligands for the immune checkpoints described above. Other mechanisms used by tumors to avoid attack include the following:

Epithelial-Mesenchymal Transition (EMT)

In this process, the cells lose their polarity and cell-cell adhesion properties and become mesenchymal stem cells that can differentiate into a variety of cell types and acquire migratory and invasive properties. A major event characterizing this transition is the loss of the cell adhesion protein E-cadherin from the cell surface. Interestingly, ß-catenin, a protein that functions both as a structural part of the cell adhesion complex and as a transcription factor, plays an important role in this process; around 10% of all tissue samples from cancers contain mutations in the ß-catenin gene. These mutations often prevent its regulated degradation, thus resulting in an accumulation of ß-catenin which translocates to the nucleus and continuously drives the transcription of its target genes. Another important player in driving EMT is TGF-ß (transforming growth factor-ß).

Transforming Growth Factor-ß (TGF-ß)

This factor often plays a major role in establishing an environment of immune suppressive cells. In normal cells, the signaling pathway of TGF-β serves to stop the cell cycle at the G1 phase. In many cancer cells, however, parts of the TGF-β signaling pathway are mutated, which allows the cancer cells to proliferate. The tumor cells induce the surrounding stromal cells (fibroblasts) to differentiate into myofibroblasts called CAFs (cancer-associated fibroblasts) and proliferate.

Excess amounts of TGF-β and other factors produced by both the tumor cells and the CAFs have an immunosuppressive effect on the surrounding cells and promote angiogenesis.

Tumor Microenvironment

A major mechanism of resistance to immunotherapy is the establishment of a highly immunosuppressive tumor microenvironment (TME) comprising regulatory T cells (Tregs), myeloid-derived suppressor cells (MDSCs), cancer-associated fibroblasts, and M2 macrophages (TAMs). In addition to TGF-ß mentioned above, tumor cells can also overexpress various other immunosuppressive cytokines including the tumor-colony stimulating factors G-CSF (granulocyte CSF) and GM-CSF (granulocyte-macrophage CSF) to create a TME of immunosuppressive and tumor-enhancing cells. For example, myeloid-derived suppressor cells (MDSCs) can infiltrate and augment the immunosuppressive environment. Macrophages, which can assume an M1 phenotype with an antitumor/pro-inflammatory function or a protumor/anti-inflammatory phenotype associated with an M2 phenotype, are polarized by the TME to the M2 phenotype. TAMs can account for up to 50% of the tumor mass and are associated with a poor prognosis in many cancers.

Indoleamine 2,3-Dioxygenase (IDO)

Another method employed by some tumors to disarm cytotoxic T cells and NK cells is to upregulate the enzyme IDO, which inhibits T/NK cells in a two-pronged attack. By catalyzing the cleavage of tryptophane, it depletes them of an essential amino acid for cell growth and proliferation. Secondly, the accumulation of the catabolic products (kynurenines) is cytotoxic for both T cells and NK cells. The overexpression of IDO has been described in a variety of human tumor cell lineages and is often associated with a poor prognosis. Overexpression of the enzymes nitric oxide synthase (NOS) and arginase-1 also deprive T cells of L-arginine.

"Don't Eat Me" Signaling by CD47

From the perspective of the immune system, tumor cells are often very similar to normal cells. They thrive best when they cease to express unusual surface antigens that raise a red flag for recognition by immune cells. On the other hand, the overexpression of some surface molecules such as ligands for the immune checkpoints described above can protect them from an immune attack. An important example is the glycoprotein CD47, which is ubiquitously expressed on the surface of all cells. It serves both as a signaling receptor for the multifunctional protein thrombospondin-1 (TSP-1) and as a ligand for the immune checkpoint signal regulatory protein-α (SIRPα) on innate immune cells such as macrophages.

Binding of CD47 to SIRPα on the surface of macrophages serves to mark the CD47+ve cells as self. They are not phagocytosed. Young erythrocytes, for example, express a large amount of CD47 on their surface. As they age, they lose more and more CD47 until they reach a point where the amount is insufficient to protect them from macrophages (see Fig. 6.4). They are then digested to make room for new red blood cells, thus ensuring that the circulation has a constant supply of fresh erythrocytes. In addition to its inhibitory action on macrophages and other antigen-presenting cells, TSP-1 signaling via CD47 on the surface of T cells and NK cells inhibits their activity. CD47 thus functions as both an innate and adaptive immune checkpoint.

Blocking of inhibitory signaling via CD47 on cytotoxic T cells has been shown to increase tumor cell killing. Monoclonal anti-CD47 antibodies have therefore been developed that block the inhibitory signals for preventing phagocytosis and killer cell activation. The results from early clinical trials look promising but have raised concerns about the side effects caused by the phagocytosis of circulating erythrocytes. Approaches are now being developed to avoid these adverse occurrences such as targeting tumor-specific epitopes on CD47 and SIRPα or by constructing bispecific antibodies targeting additional checkpoints that are only expressed together on target cells and not on erythrocytes.

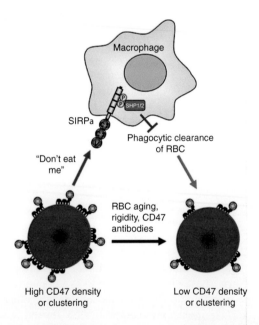

Fig. 6.4 Antiphagocytic function of CD47 on red blood cells (RBCs). Young RBCs express about 25,000 copies of CD47, which inhibits their phagocytic clearance by binding to the immune checkpoint signal regulatory protein-α (SIRPα) on macrophages. RBC aging, diseases that increase RBC rigidity, and exposure to function-blocking CD47 antibodies decrease the SIRPα-mediated "don't eat me" signal and facilitate phagocytosis. (From Kaur et al. Antibody Therapeutics (2020) **3**, 179–192; https://doi.org/10.1093/abt/tbaa017. With permission of Oxford University Press)

6.9   Hot and Cold Tumors

Antibodies against immune checkpoint inhibitors have become firmly established for the front-line treatment of some solid tumors. A significant number of complete responses in some types of solid cancer have been achieved, and they are being used for an increasing number of indications. However, most of the patients with solid tumors do not experience a long-term response. A large number of retrospective analyses have been performed to investigate which type of tumor responds best to treatment with antibodies against ICs. One of the most significant factors for a favorable outcome was the presence of tumor-infiltrating lymphocytes (TILs). These tumors typically also have a high number of mutations and have been designated as being "hot"; they include melanoma, bladder cancer, kidney cancer, head and neck cancer, and non-small cell lung cancer. Nonimmunogenic "cold" tumors such as most breast cancers, ovarian cancer, prostate cancer, pancreatic cancer, and glioblastoma have either not been infiltrated with T cells or contain only a few of them, so that it is difficult to provoke an immune response with anti-IC antibodies. Some clinical data indicate that it may be possible to convert a "cold" tumor into a "hot" tumor. The more data that can be gathered on signaling mechanisms between tumor cells and their environment, the more possibilities will be opened for recognizing potential points of attack.

Selected Literature

Akalu YT, Rothlin CV, Ghosh S. TAM receptor tyrosine kinases as emerging targets of innate immune checkpoint blockade for cancer therapy. Immunol Rev. 2017;276(1):165–77. https://doi.org/10.1111/imr.12522.

Allegra CJ, Yothers G, O'Connell MJ, et al. Phase III trial assessing bevacizumab in stages II and III carcinoma of the colon: results of NSABP protocol C-08. J Clin Oncol. 2011;29:11–6. https://doi.org/10.1200/JCO.2010.30.0855.

Baselga J, Cortés J, Kim S-B. Pertuzumab plus trastuzumab plus docetaxel for metastatic breast cancer. N Engl J Med. 2012;366(2):109–19. https://doi.org/10.1056/NEJMoa1113216.

Bonaventura P, Shekarian T, Alcazer V, et al. Cold tumors: a therapeutic challenge for immunotherapy. Front Immunol. 2019;10:168. https://doi.org/10.3389/fimmu.2019.00168.

Bridgewater JA, Pugh SA, Maishman T. Systemic chemotherapy with or without cetuximab in patients with resectable colorectal liver metastasis (new EPOC): long-term results of a multicentre, randomised, controlled, phase 3 trial. Lancet Oncol. 2020;21:398–411. https://doi.org/10.1016/S1470-2045(19)30798-3.

Campesato LF, Weng C-H, Merghoub T. Innate immune checkpoints for cancer immunotherapy: expanding the scope of non T cell targets. Ann Transl Med. 2020;8(16):1031. https://doi.org/10.21037/atm-20-1816.

Chen J, Zhong M-C, Guo H. SLAMF7 is critical for phagocytosis of haematopoietic tumour cells via mac-1 integrin. Nature. 2017;544(7651):493–7. https://doi.org/10.1038/nature22076.

Chiu ML, Goulet DR, Teplyakov A, Gilliland GL. Antibody structure and function: the basis for engineering therapeutics. Antibodies. 2019;8(4):55. https://doi.org/10.3390/antib8040055.

Coiffier B, Thieblemont C, Van Den Neste E. Long-term outcome of patients in the LNH-98.5 trial, the first randomized study comparing rituximab-CHOP to standard CHOP chemotherapy in DLBCL patients: a study by the Groupe d'Etudes des Lymphomes de l'Adulte. Blood. 2010;116(12):2040–5. https://doi.org/10.1182/blood-2010-03-276246.

Cortés J, Baselga J, Im Y-H, et al. Health-related quality-of-life assessment in CLEOPATRA, a phase III study combining pertuzumab with trastuzumab and docetaxel in metastatic breast cancer. Ann Oncol. 2013;24:2630–5. https://doi.org/10.1093/annonc/mdt274.

Dahan R, Barnhart BC, Li F, et al. Therapeutic activity of agonistic, human anti-CD40 monoclonal antibodies requires selective FcγR engagement. Cancer Cell. 2016;29(6):820–31. https://doi.org/10.1016/j.ccell.2016.05.001.

Delves PJ, Martin SJ, Burton DR, Roitt IM, et al. Roitt's essential immunology. 13th ed. Hoboken: Wiley; 2017.

Feng M, Jiang W, Kim BYS, et al. Phagocytosis checkpoints as new targets for cancer immunotherapy. Nat Rev Cancer. 2019;19(10):568–86. https://doi.org/10.1038/s41568-019-0183-z.

Galon J, Costes A, Sanchez-Cabo F. Type, density, and location of immune cells within human colorectal tumors predict clinical outcome. Science. 2006;313:1960–4. https://doi.org/10.1126/science.1129139.

Horvath CJ, Milton MN. The TeGenero incident and the Duff report conclusions: a series of unfortunate events or an avoidable event? Toxicol Pathol. 2009;37(3):372–83. https://doi.org/10.1177/0192623309332986.

Hurwitz H, Fehrenbacher L, Novotny W, et al. Bevacizumab plus irinotecan, fluorouracil, and leucovorin for metastatic colorectal cancer. N Engl J Med. 2004;350:2335–42.

Karapetis CS, Khambata-Ford S, Jonker DJ. K-ras mutations and benefit from cetuximab in advanced colorectal cancer. N Engl J Med. 2008;359:1757–65.

Kaur S, Cicalese KV, Banerjee R, Roberts DD. Preclinical and clinical development of therapeutic antibodies targeting functions of CD47 in the tumor microenvironment. Antibody Ther. 2020;3(3):179–92. https://doi.org/10.1093/abt/tbaa017.

Kim N, Kim HS. Targeting checkpoint receptors and molecules for therapeutic modulation of natural killer cells. Front Immunol. 2018;9:2041. https://doi.org/10.3389/fimmu.2018.02041.

Kumar V, Patel S, Tcyganov E, Gabrilovich DI. The nature of myeloid-derived suppressor cells in the tumor microenvironment. Trends Immunol. 2016;37(3):208–20. https://doi.org/10.1016/j.it.2016.01.004.

Larkin J, Chiarion-Sileni V, Gonzalez R, et al. Five-year survival with combined nivolumab and ipilimumab in advanced melanoma. N Engl J Med. 2019;381:1535–46. https://doi.org/10.1056/NEJMoa1910836.

Leach DR, Krummel MF, Allison JP. Enhancement of antitumor immunity by CTLA-4 blockade. Science. 1996;271:1734–6.

Little M, editor. Recombinant antibodies for immunotherapy. 1st ed. Cambridge: Cambridge University Press; 2009.

Lu R-M, Hwang Y-C, Liu I-J, et al. Development of therapeutic antibodies for the treatment of diseases. J Biomed Sci. 2020;27:1. https://doi.org/10.1186/s12929-019-0592-z.

Malfitano AM, Pisanti S, Napolitano F, et al. Tumor-associated macrophage status in cancer treatment. Cancers. 2020;12(7):1987. https://doi.org/10.3390/cancers12071987.

Marin-Acevedo JA, Soyano AE, Dholaria B, et al. Cancer immunotherapy beyond immune checkpoint inhibitors. J Hematol Oncol. 2018;11(1):8. https://doi.org/10.1186/s13045-017-0552-6.

Mlcochova J, Faltejskova-Vychytilova P, Ferracin M, et al. MicroRNA expression profiling identifies miR-31-5p/3p as associated with time to progression in wild-type RAS metastatic colorectal cancer treated with cetuximab. Oncotarget. 2015;6(36):38695–704.

Moja L, Tagliabue L, Balduzzi S, et al. Trastuzumab containing regimens for early breast cancer. Cochrane Database Syst Rev. 2012;(4):CD006243. https://doi.org/10.1002/14651858.CD006243.pub2.

Murphy K, Weaver C. Janeway's immunobiology. 9th ed. New York: WW Norton & Company; 2016.

Nishimura H, Nose M, Hiai H, Minato N, Honjo T, et al. Development of lupus-like autoimmune diseases by disruption of the PD-1 gene encoding an ITIM motif-carrying immunoreceptor. Immunity. 1999;11:141–51.

Pierpont TM, Limper CB, Richards KL. Past, present, and future of rituximab—the world's first oncology monoclonal antibody therapy. Front Oncol. 2018;8:163. https://doi.org/10.3389/fonc.2018.00163.

Qin S, Jiang J, Lu Y, et al. Emerging role of tumor cell plasticity in modifying therapeutic response. Signal Transduct Target Ther. 2020;5(1):228. https://doi.org/10.1038/s41392-020-00313-5.

Renner C. 20 years of rituximab treatment: what have we learnt? Future Oncol. 2019;15(36):4119–21.

Schumacher TN, Schreiber RD. Neoantigens in cancer immunotherapy. Science. 2015;348(6230):69–74.

Seidel JA, Otsuka A, Kabashima K. Anti-PD-1 and anti-CTLA-4 therapies in cancer: mechanisms of action, efficacy, and limitations. Front Oncol. 2018;8:86. https://doi.org/10.3389/fonc.2018.00086.

Shi R, Chai Y, Duan X, et al. The identification of a CD47-blocking "hotspot" and design of a CD47/PD-L1 dual-specific antibody with limited hemagglutination. Signal Transduct Target Ther. 2020;5:16.

Slamon DJ, Leyland-Jones B, Shak S, et al. Use of chemotherapy plus a monoclonal antibody against HER2 for metastatic breast cancer that overexpresses HER2. N Engl J Med. 2001;344(11):783–92. https://doi.org/10.1056/NEJM200103153441101.

Su S, Zhao J, Xing Y, et al. Immune checkpoint inhibition overcomes ADCP induced immunosuppression by macrophages. Cell. 2018;175:442–57. https://doi.org/10.1016/j.cell.2018.09.007.

Suntharalingam G, Perry MR, Ward S, et al. Cytokine storm in a phase 1 trial of the anti-CD28 monoclonal antibody TGN1412. N Engl J Med. 2006;355:1018–28.

Sutamtewagul G, Link BK. Novel treatment approaches and future perspectives in follicular lymphoma. Ther Adv Hematol. 2019;10:1–20. https://doi.org/10.1177/2040620718820510.

Tabernero J, Cohn AL, Obermannova R, et al. RAISE: a randomized, double-blind, multicenter phase III study of irinotecan, folinic acid, and 5-fluorouracil (FOLFIRI) plus ramucirumab (RAM) or placebo (PBO) in patients (pts) with metastatic colorectal carcinoma (CRC) progressive during or following first-line combination therapy with bevacizumab (bev), oxaliplatin (ox), and a fluoropyrimidine (fp). J Clin Oncol. 2015;33(3):512. https://doi.org/10.1200/jco.2015.33.3_suppl.512.

Tabernero J, Takayuki Y, Cohn AL, et al. Ramucirumab versus placebo in combination with second-line FOLFIRI in patients with metastatic colorectal carcinoma that progressed during or after first-line therapy with bevacizumab, oxaliplatin, and a fluoropyrimidine (RAISE): a randomised, double-blind, multicentre, phase 3 study. Lancet Oncol. 2015;16(5):499–508. https://doi.org/10.1016/S1470-2045(15)70127-0.

Tang J, Shalabi A, Hubbard-Lucey VM. Comprehensive analysis of the clinical immuno-oncology landscape. Ann Oncol. 2018;29:84–91. https://doi.org/10.1093/annonc/mdx755.

Xu W, Dong J, Zheng Y. Immune checkpoint protein VISTA regulates antitumor immunity by controlling myeloid cell–mediated inflammation and immunosuppression. Cancer Immunol Res. 2019;7:1497–510. https://doi.org/10.1158/2326-6066.CIR-18-0489.

Zahavi D, Weiner L. Monoclonal antibodies in cancer therapy. Antibodies. 2020;9:34. https://doi.org/10.3390/antib9030034.

Antibodies as Magic Bullets

7

Abstract

The concept of a "magic bullet" as first formulated by Paul Ehrlich can perhaps most readily be applied to antibodies "armed" with toxic substances or radionuclides. Most of the toxins from plants and bacteria are enzymes, a single molecule of which can catalyze thousands of reactions. In contrast, non-enzymatic reagents must be potent enough that only a few molecules are able to damage vital structures such as DNA and microtubules. Most of the current ADCs bind to the tubulin subunit of microtubules, which are the major components of the mitotic spindle, and inhibit their function in the process of cell division. Rapidly dividing cells such as tumor cells become stranded in the pre-mitotic phase of the cell cycle and eventually die. To equip antibodies with a radioactive payload, they are conjugated with cage-like complexes (chelators) that bind the positively charged ions of radioactive metals. In more recent approaches to diminish side effects, the antibody-chelate conjugates have been loaded with radionuclides after binding their target molecules in the tumor tissue.

7.1 Introduction

Around 1906 Paul Ehrlich started a project to exploit the potential of arsenical dyes for killing bacteria. Using an approach that became the basis for nearly all modern pharmaceutical research, his team attempted to optimize the biological activity of a lead compound through systematic chemical modifications. By screening a multitude of compounds, Ehrlich argued that it should be possible to identify a "magic bullet" that killed microbes but did not harm the human host. It was during this time that he coined the word "chemotherapy." The first "magic bullet" was named Salvarsan (a portmanteau for "saving arsenic") for the treatment of syphilis, which is caused by the parasitic spirochete *Treponema pallidum*. "Armed" antibodies

© The Author(s), under exclusive license to Springer Nature Switzerland AG 2021   79
M. Little, *Antibodies for Treating Cancer*,
https://doi.org/10.1007/978-3-030-72599-0_7

targeting only tumor cells fulfil the same criteria, whereby toxic substances or radionuclides are used as ammunition.

7.2   Toxins: "Shaken, Not Stirred"

On a September evening in London in 1978, Georgi Markov, award-winning Bulgarian writer, journalist, and broadcaster for the BBC World Service and other radio stations, felt a sharp pain in his thigh while waiting for a bus at Waterloo Bridge with other rush hour commuters. He looked behind him and saw a man picking an umbrella off the street. The man muttered "sorry" and hurriedly crossed the street to get into a taxi. Markov gave little thought to the seemingly trivial incident and continued on his way home. In the evening he developed a fever and was admitted to hospital where he died 4 days later at the age of 49. During the autopsy, the doctors found a small ball about 1.6 mm in diameter with two very small openings from which the phytotoxin ricin had entered his body. Markov had been the victim of a James Bond-style umbrella attack carried out by an agent of the Bulgarian secret service, probably because he had repeatedly criticized the communist leadership of his home country. The bullet was shot from the tip of an umbrella using compressed air.

Ricin is one of the most toxic proteins in nature. It is obtained from the husks of the seeds of the castor oil plant known as the "miracle tree" (*Ricinus communis*). A dose of 0.25 mg ricin or two to four seeds are sufficient to kill an adult. The protein consists of two chains (A and B). The B chain facilitates binding to the cell surface and uptake into small vesicles. Transport through the membrane of the vesicles into the cytosol is effected by the A chain. Only one molecule of the toxic A chain is enough to switch off the function of the ribosomes. If no more proteins are synthesized by the ribosomes, the cell automatically starts a suicide program (apoptosis).

7.3   Immunotoxins

To target only cancer cells, the cell-binding units of several phytotoxins such as ricin have been replaced by antibodies against tumor markers. With the first generation of ricin immunotoxins, optimal dosing was not possible due to capillary leak syndrome, a life-threatening permeability of the capillary vessels. In further developments, this undesirable side effect of ricin has been overcome to a large extent by changes in the sequence of the A chain.

Other phytotoxins that have often been used include saporin, gelonin, and American pokeweed (*Phytolacca americana*). Like ricin, they are all enzymes that deactivate ribosomes. The bacterial toxins *Pseudomonas* exotoxin, diphtheria toxin, anthrax toxin, and listeriolysin O have also been widely used. *Pseudomonas* exotoxin and diphtheria toxin both work by inactivating eukaryotic elongation factor 2, which plays an important role in the synthesis of proteins in the ribosomes. Anthrax inactivates enzymes that play a regulatory role in the transmission of signals within the cell. The toxin listeriolysin O forms pores in the cell membrane. In contrast to chemotherapy, where some tumor cells become resistant to every available chemotherapeutic agent (multidrug resistant, MDR), tumor cells do not develop a resistance to immunotoxins.

Uptake of Toxins in Cancer Cells

The effectiveness of the immunotoxins largely depends on the target molecule on the surface of the tumor cells. This molecule must enable efficient uptake of the immunotoxin. Examples are transport molecules such as the transferrin receptor, which binds transferrin-iron complexes for the cellular uptake of iron and shuttles between the cell surface and vesicles inside the cell. This is made possible by the budding of small membrane particles from the cell membrane, which are then transported into the cell interior, where they can fuse with endosomes. Because of the acidic environment of the endosomes, transferrin loses its binding capacity for iron, which then diffuses from the endosomes. The transferrin receptor with the bound transferrin is then transported back to the cell surface in small vesicles that have budded off from the endosome.

Treatment of Glioblastoma with a Transferrin Immunotoxin

The very efficient cellular uptake of transferrin inspired Richard Youle at the National Institutes of Health (United States) to combine it with diphtheria toxin to treat patients with glioblastoma, the most common malignant brain tumor in adults. Patients with this type of cancer usually die within the first year of being diagnosed. The immunotoxin was injected under pressure directly into the tumor. In a clinical phase II study to investigate the effectiveness, a long-lasting complete remission was achieved in about 10% of the patients. The therapeutic agent was then licensed to a company for further development to market approval. A series of mergers and acquisitions followed until the product was finally owned by the firm Celtic. A planned, large phase III study was started but then canceled for commercial reasons. The rights to the product have been returned to the NIH.

Lumoxiti for Treating Hairy Cell Leukemia

In contrast to the transferrin receptor, most of the proteins on the surface of tumor cells are internalized very slowly. An interesting exception is the protein CD22, which is found on the surface of normal B lymphocytes and on many leukemia and lymphoma cells. In the laboratories of Ira Pastan and Robert Kreitman at the NCI (National Cancer Institute, USA), the variable domains of an antibody against CD22 were fused with the toxic unit of the *Pseudomonas* exotoxin A to produce the immunotoxin Lumoxiti (moxetumomab pasudotox). In clinical trials, impressive results were obtained using this immunotoxin for the treatment of chemotherapy-resistant patients with hairy cell leukemia (HCL). This slow-growing cancer is characterized by B lymphocytes with a "hairy" appearance when viewed under the microscope.

Single-Arm Open-Label Pivotal Phase III Clinical Trial

The anti-CD22 immunotoxin Lumoxiti was evaluated in a single-arm open-label clinical trial with 80 chemotherapy-resistant patients at 32 centers in 14 countries. "Single arm" means that all the patients received the same treatment, and "open label" means that they all knew exactly what they were being administered. Since there was no division into a drug-treated group and a group only receiving a placebo, the results showing a beneficial effect have to be particularly convincing.

The patients received 40 µg/kg immunotoxin on days 1, 3, and 5 in 28-day cycles for up to 6 cycles. Treatment was stopped in the event of progressive disease and unacceptable toxicity or in the fortunate case of a complete response (CR) in the absence of any minimal residual disease (MRD). Of the 80 patients, 75% had already been treated with rituximab, 29% had prior rituximab combined with a purine analog, and 18% had a BRAF inhibitor (B-Raf belongs to the Raf family of growth signal transduction protein kinases). Fifty patients completed all 6 cycles, and 12 received fewer than 6 cycles due to MRD-free CR. Another 12 stopped early due to an adverse event which was treatment-related in 8 of the patients.

Thirty percent of the patients achieved a long-lasting complete response (CR), and the overall response rate (number of patients with partial or complete response to therapy) was 75%. Fortunately, as CD22 is not present in the early stages of B-cell development, normal B lymphocytes that are destroyed during this treatment can be regenerated from stem cells.

Lumoxiti was approved for treating hairy cell leukemia in 2018 and is now marketed by AstraZeneca Pharmaceuticals. A boxed warning included with the prescribing information advises healthcare professionals and patients about the risk of developing capillary leak syndrome. Symptoms include difficulty breathing, weight gain, hypotension, or swelling of the arms, legs, and/or face. There is also a risk of hemolytic uremic syndrome, a condition caused by the abnormal destruction of red blood cells.

Treatment of Solid Tumors with Immunotoxins

Because of the poor penetration of immunotoxins, patients with solid tumors have to endure several treatment cycles with relatively high dosages. Since most of the toxins are of vegetable or bacterial origin, there is a risk that the immune system could strongly react against the foreign proteins during a prolonged treatment. This can cause unpleasant side effects or result in a loss of efficacy due to the generation of neutralizing antibodies. At higher dosages, normal cells, especially in the liver and kidneys, can also be adversely affected.

In order to avoid immune reactions, the structure of some immunotoxins was made more "human" using genetic engineering. Replacing a few critical amino acids in a protein is sometimes enough to significantly reduce its immunogenic potential. Completely 100% human immunotoxins were produced through the use of human enzymes, which have a destructive effect when they are released inside the cell. Two examples are ribonucleases, which destroy RNA, and granzyme B, which induces apoptosis.

The penetration of solid tumors has been improved through the use of smaller antibody fragments. In Ira Pastan's laboratory, an immunotoxin has been developed for the treatment of various tumors that uses an Fv fragment for binding *Pseudomonas* exotoxin to the protein mesothelin. This protein is found on the cell surface of several types of cancer including breast, ovarian, pancreatic, lung, prostate, and glioblastoma. It is not expressed on normal cells except for the epithelium that lines the inner and outer surfaces of organs. However, since the cells of the epithelium are regularly replaced, the side effects can usually be kept at a tolerable level. In a phase I clinical trial, the maximum tolerated dose (MTD) for the immunotoxin LMB-100 was found to be 140 µg/kg given on days 1, 3, and 5 of a 21-day cycle. Unfortunately, the majority of patients developed antidrug antibodies after two cycles, indicating that LMB-100 has limited antitumor efficacy as a single agent. It is now being evaluated in a phase II trial for its efficacy in combination with pembrolizumab (an anti-PD-1 antibody, see Chap. 6) in patients with treatment-refractory mesothelioma and non-small cell lung cancer.

Shedding of Tumor Markers

Immunotoxins could potentially play a significant role in combination therapies since a synergistic effect between immunotoxins and chemotherapeutic agents has been found in preclinical trials. One explanation is that chemotherapy might prevent shedding of the tumor markers targeted by antibodies. Extensive antigen shedding appears to be a property of many malignant tumors, providing them with an escape mechanism from the surveillance of the immune system or from targeted immunotherapy. The extent of shedding appears to depend on the tumor marker. High shed levels, for example, have been found for the mesothelin tumor marker mentioned above in patients with an adenocarcinoma. A significant part of the shedded marker is bound by the immunotoxin, which can adversely affect its efficacy.

7.4   Antibody-Drug Conjugates (ADCs)

Immunotoxins can be produced as a single gene product by fusing the antibody gene with the toxin gene. Their enzymatic activity enables thousands of target molecules to be chemically altered by a single toxin molecule. Toxic chemical compounds, however, have to be chemically coupled to the antibody with a suitable linker to generate antibody-drug conjugates (ADCs). Since they have no enzymatic

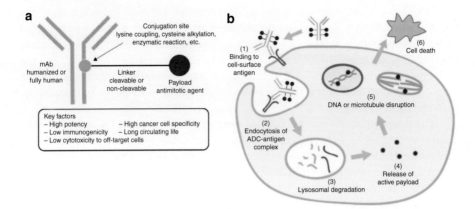

Fig. 7.1 Structure and mechanism of action of an ADC. (**a**) General structure of an ADC containing a mAb, a cleavable/non-cleavable chemical linker and a cytotoxic payload. (**b**) General mechanism of action of ADCs; binding to tumor cell target, endocytosis of the complex, lysosomal processing, release of drug into the cytosol, and disruption of DNA or microtubules. (From Tsuchikama and An. Protein Cell. (2018), **9**, 33–46. Permission for use according to creative commons license (http://creativecommons.org/licenses/by/4.0/))

activity to multiply their effect, only a few molecules must suffice to block vital structures or processes. Current ADCs act mainly by damaging DNA or by interfering with the structure of microtubules (Fig. 7.1).

ADC Conjugation

Most of the antibodies used for synthesizing ADCs are conjugated to the linker and drug payload through their lysine or cysteine residues. However, to obtain a relatively homogenous product, it is important that the drug antibody ratio (DAR) is precisely controlled to achieve a site-specific coupling of the drug payload. This has been achieved by synthesizing site-specific derivatives of the antibody before conjugation or, more recently, by protein engineering. For example, three cysteines in the antibody hinge region have been replaced with three serines leaving only two reactive cysteines, one on each chain after mild reduction, for making an ADC product with up to two molecules of drug per antibody. By refining the conditions of conjugation, it is possible to obtain ADCs containing exactly two drug molecules. Another approach for conjugation is the use of enzymes that can induce site- or amino acid sequence-specific modifications.

ADC Linker

The first generation of linkers for the connection between the toxic moiety and the antibody was not particularly stable; the conjugates could be cleaved by proteases in the circulation. As with conventional chemotherapy, the toxins that were released after linker cleavage caused adverse side effects. To avoid systemic toxicity, stable linkers were synthesized that are not cleaved by proteases before reaching their target. After internalization by a tumor cell, the antibody part of the ADCs is broken down by digestion in lysosomes, and the remaining toxic parts are released into the cytosol. To increase the efficacy of toxin release, a lot of effort was put into the development of ADCs with linkers that are not cleaved in the extracellular environment but contain sites that can be cleaved in the acidic environment of endosomes and lysosomes or by the high concentration of proteolytic enzymes in lysosomes.

Examples of ADC Linker Cleavage Sites

Hydrazone Linker
An acid-labile hydrazine group has been used for the synthesis of several ADCs. It is hydrolyzed in the acidic environment of endosomes (pH 5.0–6.0) and lysosomes (pH about 4.8). However, ADCs with a hydrazone linker also undergo a slow hydrolysis in the circulation (pH 7.4) which can limit its tolerability.

Cathepsin B Linker
Cathepsin B is a lysosomal protease that preferentially cleaves a peptide bond on the C-terminal side of sequences such as phenylalanine-lysine and valine-citrulline (Val-Cit). The cleavage efficacy can be significantly increased by combining them with *p*-aminobenzyloxycarbonyl (e.g., Val-Cit-PABC).

Disulfide Linker
This approach makes use of the much higher concentration of reducing molecules such as glutathione in the cytoplasm (1–10 mmol/L) compared to the extracellular environment (about 5 μmol/L in blood). To increase the resistance of the linker to reductive cleavage in the circulation, methyl groups are often placed next to the disulfide bond.

Drug Payloads

Many of the drugs used for making ADCs, particularly those already on the market, target microtubules. A major advantage of these drugs is that they only affect rapidly proliferating cells, such as tumor cells, by interfering with the microtubule assembly of the mitotic spindle. The cells become blocked in mitosis and eventually die. Another family of drugs used in ADCs are the highly potent DNA-damaging drugs which have potencies in the picomolar range as opposed to potencies in the nanomolar range for the tubulin-binding drugs. However, their high toxicity also means that they may significantly damage other normal cells, including stem cells, since a small portion of the drug is usually released in the circulation or the drug escapes from targeted cells (bystander effect). In the latter case, the bystander effect may also play a beneficial role by killing neighboring cells in the tumor mass that do not express the tumor target (see below).

7.5   DNA-Damaging ADCs

Mylotarg for Treating Acute Myeloid Lymphoma (AML)

The first ADC approved for clinical use in 2000 was Mylotarg (gemtuzumab ozogamicin) for the treatment of people aged over 60 years with relapsed acute myeloid leukemia (AML) who are not able to endure high-dose chemotherapy. AML is caused by a combination of mutations in the myeloblast, an immature precursor of myeloid white blood cells. The proliferation of the leukemic cells in bone marrow and blood interferes with normal blood cell production and if left untreated can be fatal within a few months. Older people who are too ill for intensive chemotherapy have a typical survival of 5–10 months.

Mylotarg comprises an IgG4 antibody targeting the cell surface protein CD33 conjugated with the extremely toxic active ingredient calicheamicin from the bacterium *Micromonospora echinospora*. CD33 is a member of the family of "siglec" proteins (sialic acid-binding immunoglobulin (Ig)-like lectins) that are abundantly expressed on hematopoietic cells, each recognizing differently linked terminal sialic acid on glycoproteins and glycolipids. It is a particularly interesting target for treating AML with ADCs since it is restricted to hematopoietic cells, where it is highly expressed on cells of myeloid lineage and quickly internalized after antigen binding. Calicheamicin binds to the minor groove of DNA and abstracts hydrogens from a deoxyribose on both strands, thereby initiating oxidative strand cleavage. A humanized IgG4 antibody was used because this class of antibody is not taken up by the neonatal receptor on the endothelium (the inner wall coating of lymph and blood vessels). Within the first year after approval, the FDA issued a black box warning on the risk of veno-occlusive disease (VOD), and in a later clinical trial, the fatal toxicity rate was significantly higher than in the standard chemotherapy group. In 2010, the FDA requested Pfizer to withdraw Mylotarg from the market. However, after a meta-analysis of prior trials and an open-label phase III trial with 280 older people, Pfizer reapplied for approval, which was granted in the United States and EU in 2017.

Besponsa for Treating Relapsed Acute Lymphoblastic Leukemia (B-ALL)

The calicheamicin-ADC Besponsa (inotuzumab ozogamicin) against the CD22 antigen was approved for the treatment of relapsed or refractory B-cell precursor acute lymphoblastic leukemia (ALL) in 2017. This cancer is characterized by a high proliferation of immature lymphocytes. If left untreated the disease progresses rapidly and is usually fatal after a few months. The rapidly internalizing antigen CD22 on B-ALL is an excellent target for treatment with ADCs (see above). Besponsa was shown to be more effective than standard chemotherapy in a clinical study involving 326 adults with CD22-positive B-cell precursor ALL, who had relapsed or had not responded to previous treatment. Patients were considered to have responded if they had no remaining cancerous B cells in their blood and bone marrow after treatment. It is given as an intravenous infusion for about 1 h on days 1, 8, and 15 of a 3- or 4-week treatment cycle. An analysis of the first 218 patients treated showed that after at least 2 cycles of treatment, 81% of patients receiving Besponsa responded to treatment compared with 29% of patients receiving standard chemotherapy. Patients who responded to treatment could proceed to have a stem cell transplant. The most common serious adverse effects ($\geq$2%) in people taking the drug in the clinical trial leading to approval were infections (23%), loss of neutrophils with fever (11%), hemorrhage (5%), stomach pain (3%), fever (3%), VOD (2%), and tiredness (2%).

In order to produce even more potent DNA-damaging ADCs, the firm Synthon developed drugs based on a new family of duocarmycin derivatives. The duocarmycins are alkylating agents originally isolated from *Streptomyces* bacteria that bind to the small groove of DNA and form a stable adduct that finally results in DNA cleavage and apoptosis. Two other highly toxic payloads that are being used for the development of ADCs are pyrrolobenzodiazepine and doxorubicin.

7.6   Microtubule Destabilizing ADCs

During the initiation of cell division (mitosis and also meiosis), a mitotic spindle is built up from microtubules to facilitate the separation of sister chromatids between the daughter cells. A microtubule has a diameter of about 25 nm and consists of 13 protofilaments of the protein tubulin. The polymerization of tubulin to a microtubule is a very dynamic process with simultaneous buildup and breakdown at both ends. The microtubules grow when the rate of tubulin uptake outweighs the rate of breakdown. Mitotic poisons such as the vinca alkaloids and taxanes bind to the ends of the microtubules and disrupt the ordered microtubule assembly process. The cell becomes locked in the mitotic phase of cell division and eventually dies.

Adcetris for Treating Hodgkin's Lymphoma

Hodgkin's lymphoma (HL) mainly involves peripheral lymph nodes and is one of the most common malignancies in young adults with a second peak in the elderly. It has a high cure rate after standard cycles of chemotherapy, but about 20–35% of the patients relapse and about half of these eventually die. HL is unusual in that the malignant cells account for only about 1–5% of the cells in the tumor tissue. Derived from a B-cell lineage, they comprise Hodgkin (H) and Reed-Sternberg (RS) cells, representing small mononucleated and large mono- or multinucleated subtypes, respectively, collectively termed Hodgkin and Reed-Sternberg (HRS) cells. Research is ongoing as to how they harness cells such as lymphocytes, monocytes, granulocytes, and fibroblasts to form the major portion of the tumor mass. The well-internalizing CD30 antigen is expressed at a high level only on HRS cells and some other lymphoid neoplasms including anaplastic large cell lymphoma (ALCL) and a subset of peripheral T-cell lymphomas.

The ADC Adcetris (brentuximab vedotin) is a chimeric anti-CD30 antigen conjugated with the microtubule inhibitor monomethyl auristatin E (MMAE) that was developed by Seattle Genetics to treat Hodgkin lymphoma (HL) and aplastic large cell lymphoma (ALCL). Adcetris showed a very high efficacy in a pivotal phase II study with relapsed or refractory HL after high-dose chemotherapy (HDC) with autologous stem cell transplant (ASCT). One hundred two patients were treated with Adcetris at a dose of 1.8 mg/kg in a 21-day cycle, for up to 16 cycles. The objective response rate (ORR, defined by the FDA as "the proportion of patients with tumor size reduction of a predefined amount and for a minimum time period") was 75% and the complete response rate was 34%. The most common adverse effect was a peripheral sensory neuropathy. Twenty patients (9 with neuropathy) discontinued because of adverse effects. Thirty-eight percent of the patients with a complete response survived without progression for more than 5 years. Based on these results, the FDA granted accelerated approval for Adcetris in 2011 for HL or ALCL that relapsed or became refractory after HDC/ASCT or for use after failure of two or more prior lines of multiagent chemotherapy in transplant-ineligible patients.

Polivy for Treating Diffuse Large B-Cell Lymphoma (DLBCL)

Diffuse large B-cell lymphoma (DLBCL) is the most common form of non-Hodgkin lymphoma accounting for about a third of all cases. Although it is a fast-growing type of NHL, which is generally responsive to standard front-line therapy, as many as 40% of the patients relapse. The ADC Polivy (polatuzumab vedotin) comprises an antibody targeting CD79b conjugated with the microtubule inhibitor monomethyl auristatin E (MMAE). It is the first commercial therapeutic ADC produced using a site-specific covalent bond conjugated to MMAE via engineered cysteines. It has been approved for use in combination with bendamustine and rituximab (BR), to treat adult patients with diffuse large B-cell lymphoma that has progressed or returned after at least two prior therapies. A complete remission was found for 40% of patients (16 out of 40) taking Polivy + BR compared to 18% taking only BR (7 out of 40). On the basis of these results, it was granted accelerated approval, but further clinical trials are required to verify and better evaluate its clinical benefit.

Kadcyla for Treating Metastatic Breast Cancer

The humanized antibody Herceptin (trastuzumab) has been conjugated with a potent derivative of maytansine (mertansine, DM1) to make the ADC Kadcyla (ado-trastuzumab emtansine) for treating breast cancer patients whose tumor cells express the HER2 growth factor. In the United States, it was specifically approved for patients who have previously been treated with Herceptin and a taxane (paclitaxel or docetaxel) and who have already been treated for metastatic breast cancer or developed tumor recurrence. In addition to the effect of naked Herceptin (see Chap. 6), the ADC has the additional toxic effect of DM1. In the EMILIA study, a phase III clinical trial compared the effect of Kadcyla versus Xeloda (capecitabine) plus Tykerb (lapatinib) in 991 people with unresectable, locally advanced or metastatic HER2-positive breast cancer who had previously been treated with Herceptin and taxane chemotherapy. This trial showed improved progression-free survival in patients treated with Kadcyla (median 9.6 vs. 6.4 months), along with improved overall survival (median 30.9 vs. 25.1 months).

Enhertu for Treating Metastatic Breast Cancer

The antibody Herceptin was conjugated with the topoisomerase I inhibitor deruxtecan to make the ADC Enhertu (trastuzumab deruxtecan) for treating adults with unresectable or metastatic HER2-positive breast cancer who have received two or more prior anti-HER2-based regimens. Its approval in the United States was based on a clinical study with 184 women who had been heavily pretreated in the metastatic setting including at least 2 anti-HER2 therapies. Enhertu was administered every 3 weeks, and the tumors were imaged every 6 weeks. The overall response rate was 60.3% (patients with measurable tumor shrinkage) with a median duration of response of 14.8 months. The prescribing information includes a black box warning for interstitial lung disease which causes scarring of lung tissues. Interstitial lung disease and pneumonitis (inflammation of lung tissue) appear to have been the cause of some fatalities.

Trodelvy for Treating Triple-Negative Breast Cancer

Triple-negative breast cancer is a type of breast cancer that tests negative for estrogen receptors, progesterone receptors, and HER2 (human epidermal growth factor receptor 2). Approximately two out of ten diagnosed breast cancers are triple-negative. The ADC Trodelvy (sacituzumab govitecan) was developed by conjugating a humanized IgG1 antibody to Trop-2 with the topoisomerase 1 inhibitor SN-38, an active metabolite of irinotecan. The Trop-2 receptor is found on many cancer cells but has only limited expression on normal cells. Trodelvy was approved for the treatment of adult patients with metastatic triple-negative breast cancer (mTNBC) who have received at least two prior therapies for metastatic disease. In a single-arm phase II study, Trodelvy demonstrated an ORR of 33.3% and a median duration of response (DoR) of 7.7 months in 108 adult TNBC patients who had previously received an average of 3 prior systemic therapies. It comes with a black box warning that it can cause severe or life-threatening neutropenia (abnormally low levels of white blood cells).

Padcev for Treating Bladder Cancer

The FDA granted accelerated approval for Padcev (enfortumab vedotin), an ADC for the treatment of advanced urothelial cancer that progressed after standard therapy and immunotherapy. It comprises a fully human IgG1 antibody directed against Nectin-4, a type I transmembrane protein receptor that is highly expressed in bladder cancer, conjugated with the monomethyl auristatin E (MMAE) microtubule inhibitor. Its effect was tested in a trial involving 125 patients with advanced urothelial carcinoma who had already been treated with platinum chemotherapy (such as cisplatin) and immunotherapy (specifically, a PD-1 or PD-L1 inhibitor, see Chap. 6). Twelve percent of the patients had a complete response and 32% a partial response. The average time for the duration of improvements was 7.6 months. Further clinical trials are required to confirm the results.

At the time of writing, *Blenrep* was the last in a steadily increasing number of ADCs to be approved for cancer therapy. Blenrep (belantamab mafodotin) is a humanized IgG1 conjugated with the microtubule inhibitor MMAF targeting BCMA (B-cell maturation antigen) for the treatment of relapsed or refractory multiple myeloma (Table 7.1).

Table 7.1 Monoclonal antibody conjugates (ADCs) approved for cancer therapy

Trade name	mAb-ADC	Format	Target	Approval	Indication of first approval (United States)
Mylotarg	Gemtuzumab ozogamicin	Humanized IgG4—calicheamicin	CD33	2000	Acute myeloid leukemia (AML)
Adcetris	Brentuximab vedotin	Chimeric IgG1—MMAE	CD30	2011	Hodgkin lymphoma
Kadcyla	Trastuzumab emtansine	Humanized IgG1—mertansine	HER2	2013	Breast cancer
Besponsa	Inotuzumab ozogamicin	Humanized IgG4—calicheamicin	CD22	2017	Acute lymphoblastic leukemia (ALL)
Polivy	Polatuzumab vedotin	Humanized IgG1—MMAE	CD79b	2019	Diffuse large B-cell lymphoma
Enhertu	Trastuzumab deruxtecan	Humanized IgG1—deruxtecan	HER2	2019	Unresectable/metastatic HER2+ve breast cancer
Trodelvy	Sacituzumab govitecan	Humanized IgG—SN-38	Trop-2 receptor	2020	Metastatic triple-negative breast cancer
Padcev	Enfortumab vedotin	Human IgG1—MMAE	Nectin-4	2020	Advanced urothelial cancer
Blenrep	Belantamab mafodotin	Humanized IgG1—MMAF	BCMA	2020	Relapsed/refractory multiple myeloma

MMAE monomethyl auristatin E, *PE38* truncated form of *Pseudomonas* exotoxin, *deruxtecan* topoisomerase 1 inhibitor, *SN-39 (active metabolite of irinotecan)* topoisomerase 1 inhibitor, *BCMA* B-cell maturation antigen, *MMAF* monomethyl auristatin F

More than 80 ADCs are now in various stages of clinical trials. This number is expected to significantly increase in the near future due to major technological improvements in linker design to increase the amount of payload and improve safety, delivery, and release. Novel toxins and modifications to existing molecules are also contributing to more effective ADCs with less side effects.

7.7   Antibody-Directed Enzyme Prodrug Therapy (ADEPT)

The prodrug concept for the treatment of cancer was first promoted by Kenneth Bagshawe at Imperial College London and then further developed at the ICL by Kerry Chester, Surinder Sharma and Richard Begent. Prodrugs are relatively harmless until they are converted into highly toxic substances by enzymatic cleavage. To selectively kill tumor cells, enzymes able to cleave the prodrug are targeted to the tumor site by fusing them with antibodies directed against tumor-associated antigens. The prodrug is administered after all of the circulating fusion protein has been removed from the circulation. This procedure became known under the acronym ADEPT (antibody-directed enzyme prodrug therapy).

In a phase I clinical study, carcinoembryonic antigen (CEA), which is often over-expressed on the tumor cells of patients with colon cancer, was targeted by the ICL scientists with an anti-CEA antibody fragment fused to carboxypeptidase G2, which was mannosylated to facilitate its clearance from normal tissue via the liver. After clearance, a bis-iodo phenol mustard prodrug was administered to patients in increasing amounts before reaching dose-limiting toxicity. However, further progress was hindered by immunogenicity problems and side effects due to the release of the toxic drug into the circulation. Various mutations were introduced to reduce the immunogenicity of the bacterial carboxypeptidase. It may be possible in future developments to use intracellular human enzymes such as β-glucuronidase for cleaving prodrugs.

7.8   Cytokine Payloads

Two cytokines, IFNα and IL-2, have been approved as monotherapies for cancer treatment, IFNα for adjuvant treatment of completely resected high-risk melanoma patients and several refractory malignancies and IL-2 for treating metastatic renal cell cancer and melanoma. The initial use of IL-2 for treating solid tumors was based on data showing that it was essential for initiating an immune response and for the proliferation of T cells. However, as is the case for most of the cytokines, it is also part of an intricate signaling system that has evolved not only to activate the immune system but also to prevent an overshooting reaction. For example, although IL-2 is essential for a cytotoxic T-cell immune response, it also stimulates Treg cells and induces the expression of immune checkpoints. Nevertheless, despite severe side effects such as capillary leak syndrome and hypotension, the administration of IL-2 is able to induce durable remissions. In a large number of clinical trials, approximately 7% of patients consistently achieved complete responses after being treated with IL-2.

The immune stimulatory effects of other cytokines such as GM-CSF, IFNγ, IL-7, IL-12, IL-21, and IL-15 have also been investigated as monotherapies in clinical trials but with largely disappointing results. They are also often associated with severe dose-limiting toxicities. A promising approach to avoid the systemic toxic effects of cytokines and achieve a tumor-specific immune response is to link them with antibodies directed against tumor-associated antigens. For example, a combination of two fusion proteins comprising IL-2 or TNFα linked to the antibody L19 which targets the fibronectin extra domain B has progressed into late-stage clinical trials for the treatment of melanoma (see Chap. 11).

7.9   Antibodies with Radioactive Payloads

In order to load antibodies with radionuclides, they are conjugated with chelating agents that strongly bind the positively charged ions of radioactive metals with negative charges. Depending on the metal, three different types of radiation are emitted:

– α-radiation, which consists of particles of two protons and two neutrons (this corresponds to the nucleus of a helium atom)
– ß-radiation, which consists of electrons
– γ-radiation, which consists of high energy photons with very short wavelengths

The relatively heavy and doubly positively charged α-particles readily collide with atoms, and their range is correspondingly short. They only penetrate a few hundredths of a millimeter into tissue—a sheet of paper is enough to intercept them. The faster ß-particles (electrons) with their single negative charge can penetrate 1–10 mm into tissue—an aluminum foil a few millimeters thick is needed to stop them. Electromagnetic γ-radiation can penetrate the body—a lead plate several centimeters thick is required to absorb a large part of the energy (Fig. 7.2).

Because of its long range, γ-radiation is not suitable for targeting and destroying a tumor using antibodies. Most clinical studies employ ß-emitters such as iodine-131 or yttrium-90 with a range of up to 1 cm. They can destroy many tumor cells through cross fire without too much damage to the surrounding tissue. The short-lived α-emitters, on the other hand, are more suitable for the treatment of small, homogeneous tumors, including leukemias, which they can destroy with high energy without significant collateral damage. However, there are some technical difficulties and stability problems that impede their use.

A major disadvantage of some α-emitters is their half-life of only a few hours, which is a logistical problem for the treatment of patients. The conjugation of an

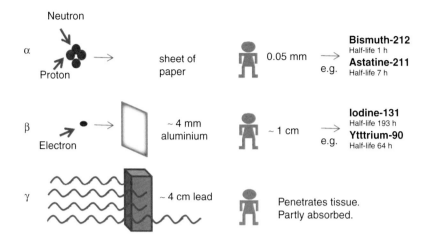

Fig. 7.2   α-, β-, and γ-radiation of radioactive atoms

antibody with a radionuclide must take place close to the treatment site, and the tumor cells must be readily accessible after administration of the radioactively loaded antibodies. Examples of suitable targets are leukemias and tumor cells in the abdominal cavity or brain cavity of a surgically removed tumor (in order to destroy any remaining tumor cells). Alternatively, the tumor cells can be pre-targeted.

Pre-targeting Tumor Cells for Radiotherapy

After an antibody is given intravenously, it can take 24 h before a significant amount accumulates in a tumor. Since antibodies are only slowly removed from the bloodstream, other tissues, especially the sensitive red bone marrow, suffer from the circulating radioactivity. To minimize background radiation and limit collateral damage, and also to facilitate a more effective employment of short-lived α-emitters, tumors can be pre-targeted with antibodies prior to delivery of a radionuclide. After the antibodies have accumulated in the tumor tissue, the radio-nuclide-chelator complexes (RCC) are injected into the bloodstream and captured by the antibodies. The small unbound RCCs are cleared relatively quickly through the kidneys.

The high affinity of some biological molecules for one another can be used to couple the radionuclide complex to the antibody. For example, the very strong binding of streptavidin or avidin with the vitamin biotin can be exploited to capture RCC-biotin conjugates with an antibody-streptavidin conjugate. To clear the unbound targeting vector from the circulation before administering the radionuclide, a biotinylated clearing agent such as albumin conjugated to galactose is often used. Since galactose has a high affinity for liver, the excess antibody-streptavidin conjugate will be removed together with the bound biotinylated albumin via hepatic

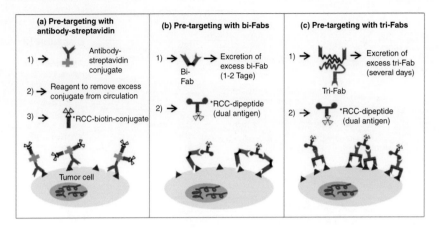

Fig. 7.3 Pre-targeting of a cancer cell for binding radionuclides. (**a**) Administration of antibody-streptavidin conjugate, which is removed from circulation with a clearing agent after accumulation in tumor, followed by administration of radionuclide complex. (**b**) Administration of bi-Fab targeting tumor antigen and peptide linked to RCC. After excretion of excess bi-Fab (1–2 days), administration of RCC-dipeptide. (**c**) Administration of tri-Fab targeting tumor antigen (bivalent binding) and peptide linked to RCC. After excretion of excess tri-Fab (several days), administration of RCC-dipeptide. *RCC radionuclide-chelator-complex

catabolism. Alternatively, smaller antibody fragments can be used that are more rapidly excreted. For example, two Fab fragments binding a tumor marker and an RCC, respectively, were linked with one another to make a bispecific molecule (Bi-Fabs). An RCC conjugated to a dipeptide comprising two identical antigens was used to improve the efficacy (see Fig. 7.3).

The latter approach was taken a step further by creating a complex of three Fab fragments using a so-called dock-and-lock technology (tri-Fabs). Two Fabs, one binding to a tumor antigen and the other to an RCC, were fused with the binding domains of the enzyme protein kinase and the protein to which it is anchored in the cell membrane, respectively. Since the binding domain of the protein kinase also binds with itself, a molecular complex is created comprising three Fabs, thus facilitating a strong binding of antibody-RCCs onto the cell surface (Fig. 7.3). The complex was further stabilized by incorporating cysteines to form disulfide bridges (locking). Several other bioconjugation methods for pre-targeting have been developed including radiolabeled complementary oligonucleotides and "click chemistry" using pairs of functional groups such as *trans*-cyclooctene and tetrazine that selectively, rapidly, and covalently bind to one another.

A disadvantage of pre-targeting is the relatively large amount of RCC required, since a significant proportion is quickly excreted through the kidneys. The amount of radioactivity in the tumor is often much lower than after treatment with antibodies that are directly conjugated with the RCC. So far, no treatment involving pre-targeting has been approved, although the technology has made significant advances in the past few years.

7.10   Radiolabeled Antibodies for Treating Follicular Lymphomas (FL)

In the United States and Europe, FLs are the second most common form of non-Hodgkin's lymphomas (NHL) after diffuse large B-cell lymphomas (DLBCL). NHLs affect the lymphatic system and disseminate to all parts of the body, for example, to lymph nodes, spleen, bone marrow, blood, and other organs where they form lymphomas, the most common form of blood cancer. About 80% of all NHL are derived from B lymphocytes and about 20% from T lymphocytes. FLs are characterized by follicle-like structures in the tissues they invade. It is a typically indolent disease, but each year 2–3% of the cases progress to a highly aggressive form.

Two antibodies conjugated with radionuclides, Zevalin and Bexxar, which bind the CD20 molecule on the surface of malignant B lymphocytes, have been approved for the treatment of indolent follicular tumors refractory to standard treatments. Both antibodies were able to destroy tumor cells that were resistant to the otherwise highly effective chimeric antibody Rituxan/MabThera (rituximab), which also binds the CD20 antigen.

Zevalin comprises the IgG1 mouse monoclonal antibody ibritumomab linked through the radionuclide-chelator tiuxetan to the β-emitter yttrium-90. Its binding domain was used for the construction of the chimeric antibody rituximab. The antibody is usually administered on an outpatient basis and comprises two treatments, approximately 1 week apart. For the first treatment, only Rituxan is administered in order to reduce the large number of B lymphocytes. A week later, the same amount of Rituxan is again administered (250 mg/m^2 intravenously) followed within 4 h by an intravenous infusion of Zevalin over 10 min at a dose of 0.3 mCi per kg (11.1 MBq per kg) with a maximum allowable dose of 32 mCi (1184 MBq).

In 2014, Zevalin received expanded approval for first-line consolidation therapy of NHL patients after initial treatment with chemotherapy based on a randomized phase III trial involving 414 patients with newly diagnosed advanced FL, which showed an improvement of median progression-free survival (PFS) of 4.1 versus 1.1 years. Consolidation therapy is a relatively intensive short-course treatment given after standard therapy that is usually limited to a high-risk population such as patients with a high FL international prognostic index (FLIPI) or patients with residual disease.

Bexxar comprises the IgG2a mouse monoclonal antibody tositumomab covalently linked through tyrosine residues to iodine-131. In contrast to the non-radioactive antibody Rituxan, which is also directed against CD20, the constant domains of Bexxar and Zevalin were not replaced by human constant domains. The risk of a severe immune reaction is relatively low since treatment with these antibodies was designed as a single application. Furthermore, murine antibodies have shorter half-lives in the circulation compared to similar antibodies with human constant domains, thus reducing damage to normal tissues by unbound antibodies. The generation of blood cells in the red bone marrow, for example, is particularly endangered by circulating radioactivity. Bexxar is administered using a similar treatment schedule to that of Zevalin except that a thyroid protective regimen begins on the first day and is continued for 14 days after therapy. The first treatment also includes a dosimetric step using a small amount of Bexxar (5 mCi) in order to study its bio-distribution. If the biodistribution is acceptable after about a week, this is followed by a therapeutic dose calculated to deliver 65 cGy of total body irradiation.

Bexxar versus Zevalin: Both have shown high efficacy in clinical studies. Unfortunately, at the time Bexxar was commercially available, no comparative studies had been carried out to help doctors and patients make decisions for choosing the most appropriate radiolabeled antibody. Considering that yttrium-90 has a range of 5–10 mm and I-131 has a range of 1–2 mm, Zevalin may be slightly better for treating larger tumors and Bexxar for treating metastases and smaller tumors. However, the longer range of Zevalin could lead to more damage to the surrounding tissue. The β-radiation from Zevalin (half-life 2.7 days) has more energy than the β-radiation from Bexxar (half-life 8 days). Since a significant part of the radiation energy of iodine-131 also comprises γ-radiation, patients are sometimes kept in quarantine for about 1–2 weeks, depending on the country.

In 2011, a comparative study with 554 patients of Rituxan and Bexxar in combination with chemotherapy showed that while both treatments gave excellent results, there was no statistical improvement for those patients treated with Bexxar. However, these results do not rule out the possibility that patients who are resistant to Rituxan would not benefit from treatment with Bexxar. Nevertheless, based on these results and the strong competition from the somewhat easier-to-administer Zevalin, GlaxoSmithKline decided to withdraw Bexxar from the market in February 2014.

Although no other radioactively labeled mAbs besides Bexxar and Zevalin have been approved for cancer therapy, recent data from some clinically advanced products look very promising. For example, a biologics license application (BLA) has been filed for the radioactively labeled murine IgG1 antibody ^{131}I-omburtamab targeting the B7-H3 antigen found on the surface of many solid tumors. It is being tested for the treatment of pediatric patients with central nervous system (CNS)/leptomeningeal metastasis from neuroblastoma. Betalutin comprising the mAb lilotomab labeled through the linker satetraxetan with the beta emitter lutetium-177 was granted fast-track status in 2020 for the treatment of relapsed or refractory marginal zone lymphoma. It is directed against the CD37 antigen found on the surface of mature B cells. Fast-track status is given to facilitate the rapid development of drugs which treat a serious or life-threatening condition and fill an unmet medical need.

Radioimmunotherapy of outpatients has not been widely adopted by the medical community due to concerns about the risk of secondary blood cancers and the availability of many competing non-radioactively labeled mAbs and small molecule products such as Imbruvica (ibrutinib) which inhibits Bruton's tyrosine kinase (BTK) in B cells. A major obstacle is probably also the inability to administer radiotherapeutics in their own departments. This is unfortunate since the radioimmunotherapy of NHL patients resistant to both chemotherapy and rituximab has been shown to be relatively safe with proven high clinical efficacy.

Treatment of Solid Tumors with Radioactively Labeled Antibodies

To date, no radioactively labeled antibodies have been approved for the treatment of solid tumors. In contrast to leukemias and lymphomas, it can take several days for solid tumors to accumulate a sufficient amount of radioactivity due to their poor permeability. During this time, the relatively high amounts of circulating radioactivity can cause significant collateral damage to normal tissues. Several approaches have therefore employed antibody fragments (see above) which can better penetrate the tumor mass. However, since the fragments are excreted relatively quickly through the kidneys, high amounts must be administered to achieve a therapeutic effect, and residual radioactive metals could cause kidney damage. A possible solution to some of these problems may be provided by the pre-targeting approaches described above. The use of alternative beta emitters, such as ^{177}Lu, ^{67}Cu, or alpha-emitters, such as ^{211}At may also help to improve the efficacy of radioimmunotherapy. Its major potential, however, may lie in its ability to kill the last remaining malignant cells and tumor stem cells at the stage of minimal residual disease after standard therapy.

Selected Literature

Akhavan D, Yazaki P, Yamauchi D, et al. Phase I study of Yttrium-90 radiolabeled M5A anti-carcinoembryonic antigen humanized antibody in patients with advanced carcinoembryonic antigen producing malignancies. Cancer Biother Radiopharm. 2020;35(1):10–5. https://doi.org/10.1089/cbr.2019.2992.

Chiu ML, Goulet DR, Teplyakov A, Gilliland GL. Antibody structure and function: the basis for engineering therapeutics. Antibodies. 2019;8(4):55. https://doi.org/10.3390/antib8040055.

Conlon KC, Miljkovic MD, Waldmann TA. Cytokines in the treatment of cancer. J Interf Cytokine Res. 2019;39(1):6–21. https://doi.org/10.1089/jir.2018.0019.

Goldenberg DM, Sharkey RM. Sacituzumab govitecan, a novel, third-generation, antibody-drug conjugate (ADC) for cancer therapy. Expert Opin Biol Ther. 2020;20(8):871–85. https://doi.org/10.1080/14712598.2020.1757067.

Guerrero-Ochoa P, Aguilar-Machado D, Ibáñez-Pérez R, et al. Production of a granulysin-based, Tn-targeted cytolytic immunotoxin using pulsed electric field technology. Int J Mol Sci. 2020;21(17):6165. https://doi.org/10.3390/ijms21176165.

Hagerty BL, Pegna GJ, Xu J, et al. Mesothelin-targeted recombinant immunotoxins for solid tumors. Biomol Ther. 2020;10(7):973. https://doi.org/10.3390/biom10070973.

Hedrich WD, Fandy TE, Ashour HM, Wang H, Hassan HE. Antibody-drug conjugates: pharmacokinetic/pharmacodynamic modeling, preclinical characterization, clinical studies, and lessons learned. Clin Pharmacokinet. 2018;57(6):687–703. https://doi.org/10.1007/s40262-017-0619-0.

Kraeber-Bodéré F, Rousseau C, Bodet-Milin C, et al. Tumor immunotargeting using innovative radionuclides. Int J Mol Sci. 2015;16:3932–54. https://doi.org/10.3390/ijms16023932.

Kreitman RJ. Hairy cell leukemia: present and future directions. Leuk Lymphoma. 2019;60(12):2869–79. https://doi.org/10.1080/10428194.2019.1608536.

Kreitman RJ, Pastan I. Development of recombinant immunotoxins for hairy cell leukemia. Biomol Ther. 2020;10(8):1140. https://doi.org/10.3390/biom10081140.

Leung D, Wurst JM, Liu T, et al. Antibody conjugates—recent advances and future innovations. Antibodies. 2020;9(1):2. https://doi.org/10.3390/antib9010002.

Makita S, Maruyama D, Tobinai K. Safety and efficacy of brentuximab vedotin in the treatment of classic Hodgkin lymphoma. Onco Targets Ther. 2020;13:5993–6009. https://doi.org/10.2147/OTT.S193951.

Murer P, Neri D. Antibody-cytokine fusion proteins: a novel class of biopharmaceuticals for the therapy of cancer and of chronic inflammation. New Biotechnol. 2019;52:42–53. https://doi.org/10.1016/j.nbt.2019.04.002.

Norsworthy KJ, Ko CW, Lee JE, et al. FDA approval summary: Mylotarg for treatment of patients with relapsed or refractory CD33-positive acute myeloid leukemia. Oncologist. 2018;23(9):1103–8. https://doi.org/10.1634/theoncologist.2017-0604.

Ponziani S, Di Vittorio G, Pitari G, et al. Antibody-drug conjugates: the new frontier of chemotherapy. Int J Mol Sci. 2020;21:5510. https://doi.org/10.3390/ijms21155510.

Rosenberg SA. IL-2: the first effective immunotherapy for human cancer. J Immunol. 2014;192(12):5451–8. https://doi.org/10.4049/jimmunol.1490019.

Rosenberg JE, O'Donnell PH, Balar AV, et al. Pivotal trial of enfortumab vedotin in urothelial carcinoma after platinum and anti-programmed death 1/programmed death ligand 1 therapy. J Clin Oncol. 2019;37(29):2592–600. https://doi.org/10.1200/JCO.19.01140.

Sachpekidis C, Jackson DB, Soldatos TG. Radioimmunotherapy in non-Hodgkin's lymphoma: retrospective adverse event profiling of Zevalin and Bexxar. Pharmaceuticals. 2019;12(4):141. https://doi.org/10.3390/ph12040141.

Sharkey RM, Goldenberg DM. Cancer radioimmunotherapy. Immunotherapy. 2011;3:349–70.

Sharma SK, Bagshawe KD. Antibody directed enzyme prodrug therapy (ADEPT): trials and tribulations. Adv Drug Deliv Rev. 2017;118:2–7.

Shim H. Bispecific antibodies and antibody-drug conjugates for cancer therapy: technological considerations. Biomol Ther. 2020;10(3):360. https://doi.org/10.3390/biom10030360.

Staudacher AH, Brown MP. Antibody drug conjugates and bystander killing: is antigen-dependent internalisation required? Br J Cancer. 2017;117(12):1736–42. https://doi.org/10.1038/bjc.2017.367.

Sutamtewagul G, Link BK. Novel treatment approaches and future perspectives in follicular lymphoma. Ther Adv Hematol. 2019;10:1–20. https://doi.org/10.1177/2040620718820510.

Tsuchikama K, An Z. Antibody-drug conjugates: recent advances in conjugation and linker chemistries. Protein Cell. 2018;9(1):33–46.

Verhoeven M, Seimbille Y, Dalm SU. Therapeutic applications of pretargeting. Pharmaceutics. 2019;11(9):434. https://doi.org/10.3390/pharmaceutics11090434.

Zhang Y, Pastan I. High shed antigen levels within tumors: an additional barrier to immunoconjugate therapy. Clin Cancer Res. 2008;14:7981–6.

Novel Modular Antibodies

8

Abstract

An antibody can be regarded as a modular arrangement of domains, each of which comprises the typical immunoglobulin fold, a sandwich-like structure of two β-pleated sheets stabilized by a disulfide bridge. The variable domains at the end of the Fab arms containing the hypervariable antigen-binding regions can be used for constructing "mini-antibodies" which retain the binding properties of the original antibody but without its effector functions. Alternatively, non-immunoglobulin domains of other proteins containing binding sites on a stable scaffold have also been used for creating libraries of novel binding modules. Mini-antibodies can be coupled with radioactive or other markers for diagnostic purposes, since their small size facilitates the penetration of tumor tissue. For tumor therapy, they can be coupled with other modules that provide effector functions or with the binding domains of other antibodies to make bispecific or even multispecific recombinant antibodies. For example, dual binding antibodies can be used to recruit immune cells for inducing the lysis of tumor cells. To avoid the rapid excretion of these relatively small fragments from the circulation, they can be fused with other molecules such as albumin that have a relatively long half-life.

8.1   Introduction

In 1972, the group of David Givol at the Weizmann Institute of Science in Rehovot, Israel, split the Fab′-fragment of a mouse IgA myeloma antibody directed against the hapten 2,4-dinitrophenyl with pepsin into fragments comprising variable and constant domains, respectively. The Fv fragment containing the variable domains was approximately half the size of the Fab′ fragment but had the same antigen-binding affinity. This was the first direct evidence that only the variable domains bind antigen without the participation of the constant domains. Antibody variable domains, either alone or in combination with other antibody and protein domains, have since been used for the creation of a large number of novel antibodies designed for the optimization of a particular diagnostic or therapeutic function.

8.2   Single-Chain Fv Antibodies (scFv)

The use of pepsin to obtain Fv fragments did not prove to be generally applicable. Jim Huston and his team at the firm Creative Biomolecules and the Massachusetts General Hospital and Harvard Medical School in Boston therefore designed a recombinant protein comprising the variable domains of the anti-digoxin mAb 26-10 joined by a peptide linker to avoid potential refolding problems of a two-chain fragment and also to provide more stability. X-ray data indicated that the distance between the C-terminus of the VH domain and the N-terminus of the VL domain was about 3.5 nm which should easily be bridged by a 15-residue linker with a peptide unit length of about 0.38 nm. The criteria for the linker were that it should not exhibit a propensity for ordered secondary structure or any tendency to interfere with protein folding. The 15-residue sequence (Gly-Gly-Gly-Gly-Ser)$_3$ appeared to fulfil these requirements (Fig. 8.1).

In contrast to a Fab fragment, which is stabilized by an interchain disulfide bridge and non-covalent binding between four domains (VH/VL, CH/CL), the stability of an scFv is dependent on the strength of the non-covalent binding between the VH and VL domains. Some laboratories therefore prefer to use scFvs that have been additionally stabilized by engineering an interdomain disulfide bridge or through the insertion of charged amino acids in complementary positions on the VH and VL domains to make an electrostatic bond.

Small antibody fragments such as scFvs can be produced in bacteria using expression plasmids. After the antibody gene sequence has been incorporated into the plasmid, it can be transferred into bacteria by treatment with salts (e.g., calcium chloride) and/or heat shock or, even more effectively, by an electric shock. Larger

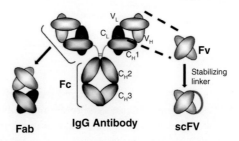

Fig. 8.1 Modular structure of an antibody. In contrast to the Fv fragment, the Fab fragment is quite stable. A peptide linker placed between the two variable domains serves to enhance the folding and stability of this small binding unit. The two domains are now on a single protein chain (*scFv* "single-chain" Fv)

antibody fragments are best produced in eukaryotic cells—the most widely used cell line is derived from the ovaries of the Chinese hamster (CHO cell, see Chap. 5).

8.3   Modular Multivalent Antibodies

The modular structure of an antibody facilitates the addition of further domains either adjacent to the variable domains at the top of the molecule or to the constant domains at the bottom end of the molecule. For example, variable domains with the same or a second antigen specificity can be fused to the end of the Fab arms to create an antibody with a total of four binding sites. Alternatively, each of the antibody variable domains can be exchanged for an scFv unit (Fig. 8.2). The larger the molecule, however, the more difficult it is to produce them in sufficiently large quantities. Smaller molecules with multiple binding sites may therefore be preferred. For example, in the examples shown in Fig. 8.2, scFvs have been fused with Fab fragments or with other scFvs. Approximately 100 such modular antibodies have already been synthesized, and many more combinations are possible. They have been referred to as a "zoo" by Brinkmann and Kontermann. Some of the species in the zoo look nice, but they can be poorly behaved and difficult to handle. Above all, they need to be druggable. This means that it must be possible to produce them economically and reproducibly in large quantities without the presence of undesired side products. They must also be thermally stable, not aggregate, and able to be stably formulated at fairly high concentrations for clinical use.

8.4   The Diabody Structure

As already described above, single-chain antibodies (scFv) are generated by connecting the VH and VL domains with a peptide linker. An important prerequisite is that the linker is long enough to enable the pairing of the two domains at the interface. If the linker is shortened, the two domains cannot come together. However, the VH and VL domains can pair with the free domains of neighboring molecules to

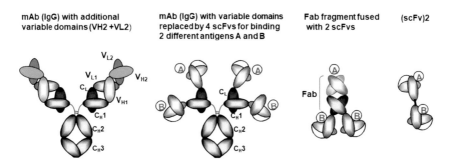

Fig. 8.2 Modular structure of some multivalent and dual binding antibodies

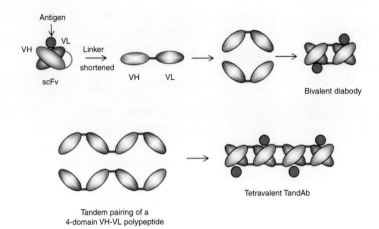

Fig. 8.3 Modular construction of a diabody. VH and VL domains joined by a linker containing less than ten amino acids do not have enough freedom of movement to bind at the VH/VL interface. However, they can form pairs with the free domains of neighboring molecules to form bivalent diabodies. Similarly, tandem pairing of a VH-VL 4-domain polypeptide occurs when the linkers are too short for internal domain pairing. This results in the formation of a so-called tetravalent TandAb (tandem diabody)

form a bivalent diabody (Fig. 8.3). Since they have an additional pair of interacting domains compared to an scFv, they are also more stable. The firm MacroGenics has increased the stability of diabodies still further by introducing cysteines at the end of the VH domains to facilitate the formation of interchain disulfide bonds. This diabody format is known as a DART (dual-affinity re-targeting). To increase the half-life in the circulation, DARTs have been fused with Fcγ domains. The diabody structure can also be stabilized by making single-chain diabodies comprised of four domains with a flexible linker in the middle to allow the four domains to fold over on themselves, generating a single-chain diabody. To avoid a rapid renal excretion of these relatively small molecules, scientists at the German Cancer Research Center in Heidelberg created a diabody format called a TandAb comprising a chain of four variable domains joined by short peptide linkers. Since the central linker is too short to permit the molecule to fold over on itself, the four domains partner with the corresponding domains of another (identical) chain to form a tetravalent molecule comprising four VH/VL units (Fig. 8.3).

8.5   Single-Domain Antibodies (sdAb) from Sharks, Camels, and Humans

Shark antibodies do not have light chains. They consist of two identical heavy chains (homodimers) each with five constant domains and one variable domain (called V-NAR, "*n*ew *a*ntigen *r*eceptor"; Fig. 8.4). Much later in evolution, the camelid family (camels, llamas, etc.) also produced homodimer antibodies, each chain

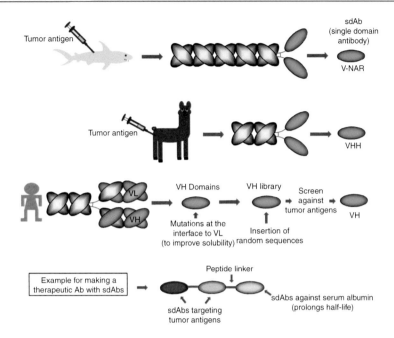

Fig. 8.4 Single-domain antibodies (sdAbs). Sharks and llamas have antibodies that contain single binding domains (*colored green*). After immunization with tumor antigens and isolation of the VH-DNA from the mRNA of B lymphocytes, these domains can be used for the production of a therapeutic sdAb (see example in lower part of figure). In contrast, the binding site of a human antibody is always formed by two different binding domains, VH and VL. Both domains can be produced as soluble single domains by introducing hydrophilic amino acid residues at the VH/VL interface. Specific VH domains against a particular antigen are obtained by screening large libraries of VH domains generated by the introduction of randomized amino acid sequences into the hypervariable regions

comprising two constant domains and one variable VH domain, in addition to the classic antibodies. After sharks or camelids have been vaccinated with antigens, specific sdAbs (also referred to as "nanobodies") can be obtained by transcribing and cloning the VH-DNA from the mRNA of B lymphocytes to make libraries of sdAbs that can be screened for the best binders using phage display (see Chap. 5).

To reduce the risk of an immune reaction, sdAbs have also been generated from the VH domains of human antibodies (Fig. 8.4), which appear to play a larger role than VL domains in binding antigens. However, without the VL domain to shield the hydrophobic VH/VL interface from the hydrophilic medium, the VH domains have a strong tendency to aggregate. This problem was solved by exchanging hydrophobic amino acid residues at the VH/VL interface for hydrophilic amino acid residues.

Since humans for ethical reasons cannot be immunized, large antibody libraries from human sdAbs have been generated by the insertion of randomized sequences into the hypervariable regions, and specific antibodies against a particular antigen have been selected by phage display as described in Chap. 5. The larger the library, the greater the chances of finding an antibody with the desired binding properties.

8.6   Binding Modules Comprising Non-Ig Protein Scaffolds: Antibody Mimetics

In principle, sdAbs can be produced on the basis of other human proteins that have no resemblance to the structure of classical antibodies. What is needed is a stable scaffold that carries a group of exposed amino acids whose sequence can be changed without affecting the stability of the scaffold. By incorporating random sequences at these exposed positions, large libraries of synthetic sequences can be made which, like the synthetic VH libraries, can be selected for binders against particular antigens.

Antibody mimetics can avoid the disadvantages often encountered with regular mAbs and their derivatives such as the high costs of production, their relatively large size, low thermostability, and storage problems in challenging environments. Currently, more than 25 different non-Ig scaffolds comprising α-helices, β-sheets, or random coils, many of them from human proteins, have been used to incorporate libraries of binding molecules generated by directed or random mutagenesis. However, whereas scaffolds from human proteins are not expected to be immunogenic, the random mutations in the binding sites might be recognized as neoantigens and provoke an immune reaction. 3D structures of eight well-known examples are shown in Fig. 8.5.

Adnectins: Derived from the tenth extracellular domain of human fibronectin type III protein comprising seven ß-strands linked by six loops, thus resembling the variable domain of an antibody (Fig. 8.5a). Libraries of adnectins have been constructed by randomizing amino acids positions in three of the CDR-like loops.

Anticalins: Derived from human lipocalins, a family of proteins that transport small hydrophobic molecules such as steroids and lipids. These 20 kDa proteins have a barrel structure formed by eight antiparallel β-strands connected by loops and an attached α-helix (Fig. 8.5b). Four exposed loops connecting the ß-strands are used for introducing random mutations.

Avimers: Derived from the A domain of extracellular receptors. The avimer domain is relatively small (4 kDa) and very resistant to thermal denaturation due to three stabilizing intradomain disulfide bridges (Fig. 8.5c). Avimer domains binding different antigens on the same protein can be linked together with small peptide linkers to obtain high-avidity binders (*avidity multimers*).

Fynomers: Derived from the human Src homology domain 3 (SH3) of the human Fyn tyrosine kinase. These small non-immunogenic globular proteins (7 kDa) contain two antiparallel ß-sheets and two flexible loops which can be used for inserting random sequences of amino acids (Fig. 8.5d). They have a high thermal stability and can easily be expressed in bacteria.

Kunitz domains: Derived from Kunitz-type protease inhibitors. They are composed of a twisted two-stranded antiparallel ß-sheet and two a-helices stabilized by

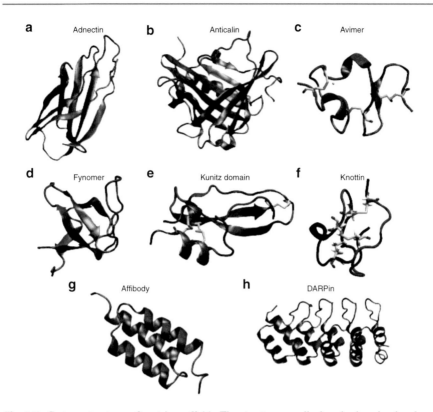

Fig. 8.5 Cartoon structures of protein scaffolds. The structures are displayed using visual molecular dynamics (VMD). The loops that recognize the antigen are colored red and the framework residues are gray. Disulfide bridges are indicated by yellow sticks and the calcium is a blue sphere. Protein scaffolds can be divided into two general categories: (1) scaffolds with ligand-binding amino acids in exposed loops (**a–f**) and (2) those with ligand-binding amino acids scattered in secondary structural motifs, e.g., α-helices (**g, h**). (From Simeon R and Chen Z. Protein Cell. 2018, **9**, 3-14. doi: https://doi.org/10.1007/s13238-017-0386-6. Permission for use according to creative commons license (http://creativecommons.org/licenses/by/4.0/))

three pairs of disulfide bonds (Fig. 8.5e). Residues in the three loops can be mutated without loss of stability.

Knottins: Thirty amino-acid (<4 dKa) protein folds of three anti-parallel ß-strands connected by loops of variable length which can be used for inserting random mutations (Fig. 8.5f). They are extremely thermostable and highly resistant to proteolysis. Their unique characteristic is a cysteine knot across a disulfide-stabilized macrocycle.

Affibodies: This 6 kDa α-helical scaffold is derived from the B domain of staphylococcal protein A (SPA). Affibodies possess the structural stability and rapid folding of the parental protein with enhanced chemical and thermal stability. Thirteen positions on two of the helices comprising the binding site were randomized for the selection of high-affinity binders to various proteins and peptides (Fig. 8.5g). They are widely used in diagnostics and are being developed for tumor imaging.

DARPins: Based on ankyrin repeat (AR) proteins which mediate various protein interactions (*designed ankyrin repeat proteins*). They contain two to three internal ARs sandwiched between the N- and C-terminal capping repeats (Fig. 8.5h). Each repeat contains a β-turn followed by two antiparallel α-helices and an unstructured loop. Random mutations can be inserted into ß-turns and the loop for generating libraries of DARPins. They are resistant to proteolysis and very thermostable and can be produced in large quantities in *E. coli*. An interesting characteristic of DARPins is their relatively large binding interface.

8.7   Size Matters

For some therapeutic applications such as the penetration of solid tumors and the delivery of toxins or radioactive payloads, the small size (2–15 kDa) of binding modules such as sdAbs, scFvs, and antibody mimetics may be an advantage. They have also proved to be extremely useful for diagnostics and tumor imaging or for intraocular treatment of the wet form of macular degeneration.

In general, however, proteins less than 50 kDa pass unhindered through the kidneys and disappear relatively quickly from the bloodstream. The small binding modules are therefore not very suitable for therapeutic use, even if two or more are fused together. One way to prevent their excretion is to fuse them with proteins such as albumin or with modified Fc domains, which have a relatively long half-life. Alternatively, they can be fused with another module that binds such proteins (Fig. 8.4).

A more detailed description of molecular formats used for making bispecific therapeutic antibodies to treat cancers is given in the following chapter.

Selected Literature

Brinkmann U, Kontermann RE. The making of bispecific antibodies. MAbs. 2017;9(2):182–212. https://doi.org/10.1080/19420862.2016.1268307.

Huston JS, Levinson D, Mudgett-Hunter M, et al. Protein engineering of antibody binding sites: recovery of specific activity in an anti-digoxin single-chain Fv analogue produced in Escherichia coli. Proc Natl Acad Sci U S A. 1988;85(16):5879–83. https://doi.org/10.1073/pnas.85.16.5879.

Inbar D, Hochman J, Givol D. Localization of antibody-combining sites within the variable portions of heavy and light chains. Proc Natl Acad Sci U S A. 1972;69(9):2659–62. https://doi.org/10.1073/pnas.69.9.2659.

Konning D, Zielonka S, Grzeschik J, et al. Camelid and shark single domain antibodies: structural features and therapeutic potential. Curr Opin Struct Biol. 2017;45:10–6. https://doi.org/10.1016/j.sbi.2016.10.019.

Simeon R, Chen Z. In vitro-engineered non-antibody protein therapeutics. Protein Cell. 2018;9(1):3–14. https://doi.org/10.1007/s13238-017-0386-6.

Spiess C, Zhai Q, Carter PJ. Alternative molecular formats and therapeutic applications for bispecific antibodies. Mol Immunol. 2015;67:95–106. https://doi.org/10.1016/j.molimm.2015.01.003.

Wang Q, Chen Y, Park J, et al. Design and production of bispecific antibodies. Antibodies (Basel). 2019;8(3):43. https://doi.org/10.3390/antib8030043.

Yu X, Yang YP, Dikici E, et al. Beyond antibodies as binding partners: the role of antibody mimetics in bioanalysis. Annu Rev Anal Chem. 2017;10(1):293–320. https://doi.org/10.1146/annurev-anchem-061516-045205.

Zielonka S, Empting M, Grzeschik J, et al. Structural insights and biomedical potential of IgNAR scaffolds from sharks. MAbs. 2015;7(1):15–25. https://doi.org/10.4161/19420862.2015.989032.

Recruiting Killer Cells for Cancer Therapy

9

Abstract

To recruit immune killer cells for treating cancer, bispecific antibodies have been developed that bind to activating receptors on the cell surface of NK and T cells and to tumor-associated antigens (TAAs). Some are based on multivalent full-length antibodies, and others comprise only single chains of antibody variable domains. Indeed, the most successful bispecific antibody to date, a so-called BiTE for treating refractory or relapsed B-cell acute lymphoblastic leukemia (B-ALL), was constructed by linking an anti-CD3 scFv to an anti-CD19 scFv for treating B-cell malignancies. Strategies to prolong the half-life of such small constructs include fusions with albumin or with modified antibody Fc domains. In a second approach, T cells were transfected with a viral vector containing a gene cassette encoding a chimeric antigen receptor (CAR). Two such chimeric antigen receptor T cells (CAR-T cells), namely, Kymriah and Yescarta targeting CD19, achieved a high number of complete responses in the treatment of refractory or relapsed B-ALL and diffuse large B-cell lymphoma (DLBCL). An increasing number of novel strategies are being developed to optimize CAR-T cell efficacy and overcome the immunosuppressive effect of the tumor microenvironment. Progress has also been made in the development of off-the-shelf allogenic products, which would not only be much cheaper but also be more widely available. A major goal of both approaches is to develop products that reduce the risk of serious adverse events due to cytokine-related syndrome (CRS) and neurotoxicity while maintaining therapeutic efficacy.

9.1   Introduction

When foreign or mutated peptides are detected by T cells or deviations in surface markers are encountered by NK cells, the aberrant cell is forced to commit suicide (apoptosis). Two major mechanisms can be employed to induce apoptosis: the activation of the Fas death receptor or the secretion of granzyme (see Chap. 2). However, the Fas-FasL pathway seems to be mainly used for controlling the effector T-cell population in a process known as activation-induced cell death (AICD), and aberrant cells are usually lysed via granzyme. To evade being attacked by immune cells, tumor cells have developed various escape mechanisms as described in Chap. 6. Methods have therefore been devised employing bispecific antibodies and chimeric antibody receptors (CARs) that link and activate cytotoxic T cells and NK cells directly with a tumor-associated antigen. In the activated killer cells, granular vesicles are transported to the cell surface where they release perforin and granzyme. Perforin interacts with the cell membrane to facilitate the entry of granzyme into the targeted cell, which then initiates a cascade of enzyme activations (the caspase cascade) resulting in proteolytic cell lysis.

9.2   Recruitment of Killer Cells with Bispecific Antibodies

Quadromas

To recruit killer cells for lysing tumor cells, bispecific antibodies have been developed that have one or more binding sites for tumor-associated antigens (TAAs) on the cancer cell and one or more binding sites for activating molecules on the surface of the killer cell. The CD3 component of the T-cell receptor (TCR) on T cells and FcγIIIA (CD16A) on NK cells are usually chosen, since they generate particularly strong activating signals.

The first bispecific antibodies were produced by chemically coupling two monoclonal antibodies. But it was very difficult to produce a homogeneous product. In a second approach, two hybridomas, each secreting murine monoclonal antibodies with different specificities, were fused with one another to create a so-called quadroma. In this cell line, the heavy and light chains of the two antibodies are randomly paired with one another, resulting in ten different antibody combinations. Since they all have the same size and fairly similar chemical compositions, it was very difficult to isolate and purify the desired bispecific combination.

Another problem using conventional monoclonal antibodies is the binding site for NK cells in the Fc domain. Antibodies with binding sites in the variable domains for T cells or for NK cells can cross-link T cells with NK cells or NK cells with other NK cells: a potentially dangerous situation that could initiate a cytokine storm. To avoid this danger, bispecific antibodies were constructed without the inherent binding site for NK cells by chemically linking two Fab fragments. Another elegant procedure to construct bispecific antibodies by non-covalently binding a total of three Fab fragments by the "dock-and-lock" method was described in Chap. 7 (Fig. 7.3) for delivering radioactive payloads to cancer cells.

Removab (Catumaxomab)

Removab was developed for treating malignant ascites in patients with EpCAM-positive cancers. It was the first bispecific antibody to be approved for cancer therapy (by the European Medicines Agency (EMA) in 2009). It was constructed by hybridizing a hybridoma secreting a murine anti-EpCAM IgG2a mAb with a hybridoma secreting a rat anti-CD3 IgG2b mAb. The isolation of the correct heterodimeric molecule was easier than usual since the rat L-chains and the mouse L-chains preferentially associated with their corresponding rat and mouse heavy chains. Removab can be regarded as a trifunctional antibody since it binds to EpCAM with one arm of the mAb, to CD3 with the other arm, and to NK cells with its Fc domain. As mentioned above, this may result in improved efficacy under certain conditions, but its potential ability to cross-link T cells and NK cells with one another could unleash a cytokine storm. However, the main issue prohibiting its systemic application appears to be the immunogenicity of the murine/rat amino acid sequences. In one clinical trial, fatal acute liver failure and cytokine release-associated toxicity were observed. Administration of catumaxomab is therefore limited to localized intraperitoneal injection. Due to commercial reasons, it was removed from the market in 2017.

9.3   Methods to Facilitate Desired Chain Pairing

A major problem with the generation of bispecific full-length human mAbs from quadromas is the purification of the correct combination of heavy and light chains. This problem was partially resolved by facilitating the desired heavy chain heterodimerization with a "knobs-into-holes" technology (Fig. 9.1). Mutations were introduced into the two CH3 domains that enabled large amino acid side chains from one CH3 domain to fit into a complementary space in the other CH3 domain. Several other asymmetric heavy chain approaches have also been employed including complementary electrostatic pairing, the use of hybrid CH3 domains from IgG and IgA and the use of antibody structure algorithms to identify those mutations that weaken homodimers and strengthen heterodimers. There remained, however, the problem of the light chains, which randomly paired with the two heavy chains of the heterodimer.

One approach to the light chain problem was to use the same light chain, since it was reasoned that very often most of the binding affinity and specificity was provided by the complementary determining regions (CDRs) of the heavy chain variable domain. However, the light chain does seem to make an important contribution to the binding properties of many antibodies. One solution to this problem was provided by the CrossMAb technology where correct pairing is achieved

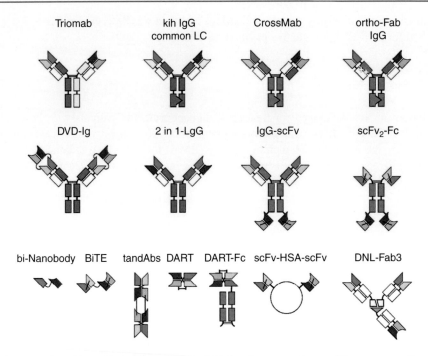

Fig. 9.1 Bispecific antibody formats in development for cancer therapy. The upper two lines depict bsAbs incorporating an IgG Fc region, either as bivalent or tetravalent molecules. Several small bsAbs and bsAb fusion proteins have entered clinical trials, and a BiTE bsAb has been approved. *BiTE* bispecific T-cell engager, *DART* dual-affinity re-targeting, *DNL* dock-and-lock, *DVD-Ig* dual variable domain immunoglobulins, *HSA* human serum albumin, *kih* knobs into holes. (From Kontermann R and Brinkmann U. Drug Discov Today 2015; 20:838–47 with permission of Elsevier)

by exchanging the CH1 domain of one heavy chain with the constant domain of the light chain (CL). For example, one arm of the CrossMAb vanucizumab binds angiopoietin-2 (Ang2) and the other arm is derived from Avastin and binds to vascular endothelial growth factor A (VEGF-A). The antibody was designed to have improved efficacy for inhibiting the tumor blood supply compared to Avastin alone. Another more recent solution has been to introduce mutations into both the CH1-CL and VH-VL interfaces that enforce the correct pairing of the light chains with the corresponding heavy chains to create a so-called orthogonal Fab interface (Fig. 9.1).

9.4   Addition of Binding Domains to Heavy and Light Chains

To avoid the difficulties of making full-length bispecific mAbs incurred by hybridization, double variable domain (DVD-Igs) antibodies have been generated by adding a second variable heavy chain domain to the heavy chain and a corresponding second variable light chain domain to the light chain of a monoclonal antibody.

Alternatively, single-chain antibodies can be fused to the C-terminal end of the antibody heavy chain. Another approach uses only the Fc domain to create tetravalent bispecific antibodies by adding single-chain antibodies to both the N-terminus and the C-terminus (Fig. 9.1). The advantage of incorporating Fc domains in bispecific antibody constructs is that they include additional effector functions including a long half-life provided by the recycling function of FcRn. However, as discussed above, binding of the Fc domain to other immune cells could be detrimental, and mutations have been identified that can remove these functions without disturbing the FcRn recycling function.

9.5   Two-in-One Antibodies

Two interesting alternative methods for the production of bispecific antibodies were developed at Genentech and at the Scripps Research Institute (San Diego). The binding site of the Herceptin blockbuster for the treatment of breast cancer was genetically engineered to create a second binding site for VEGF (vascular endothelial growth factor) in addition to the binding site for the growth factor HER2. Since VEGF stimulates the growth of blood vessels essential for the tumor, this antibody may provide a means of increasing the efficacy of treating breast cancer. Other so-called "two-in-one" antibodies are being developed in Genentech's laboratories.

9.6   Peptide-Fused Antibodies

In a quite different approach to block tumor growth factors, research scientists at the Scripps Research Institute have used antibodies as carriers of small peptides that bind to growth hormone receptors and thereby block the binding sites for the corresponding growth factor. By this means they can target receptors on the tumor cell surface with high-affinity blocking peptides carried by full-length antibodies, thus benefiting from the properties of the carrier antibody such as a long half-life and its effector functions for mediating ADCC and CDS. This technology was further developed by CovX Pharmaceuticals and then acquired by Pfizer.

9.7   Bispecific Antibodies Comprising Chains of Antibody Variable Domains

To facilitate the production of homogenous bispecific antibodies without Fc domains, single-chain gene products comprising only antibody variable domains have been constructed that fold to form bivalent and multivalent formats as described in Chap. 8. For example, the recruitment and activation of T cells and NK cells, respectively (Fig. 9.2), are shown with (a) a BiTE (bispecific T-cell engager) antibody comprising a single-chain antibody (scFv) against the CD19 antigen on malignant B lymphocytes linked by a five-amino-acid peptide to another scFv against the

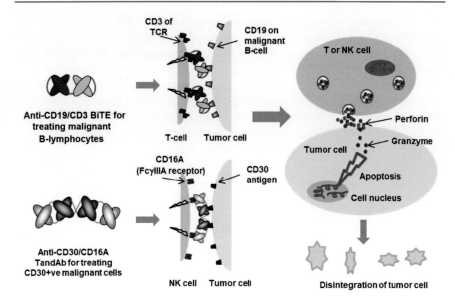

Fig. 9.2 Bispecific antibodies comprised only of antibody variable domains. Bispecific single-chain antibody (BiTE) and bispecific tetravalent TandAb for the recruitment of T and NK cells, respectively, to lyse malignant B lymphocytes or CD30+ v malignant cells such as Hodgkin lymphoma. The binding of the CD3 component of the T-cell receptor on T cells or CD16A on NK cells induces a strong activation signal resulting in the transport of granules containing perforin and granzyme to the cell surface, where the contents are released. Perforin interacts with the cell membrane to facilitate the entry of granzyme into the cell where it initiates a cascade of further enzymes (caspases) that initiate programmed cell death (apoptosis)

CD3ε component of the T-cell receptor (TCR) and (b) a TandAb (tandem antibody) comprising a chain of four antibody variable domains which dimerizes with itself to form two binding VH/VL units directed against the CD30 antigen on the surface of Hodgkin lymphoma and two VH/VL units directed against FcγRIIIA (CD16A) on NK cells.

Blincyto (Blinatumomab) for Treating Acute Lymphoblastic Leukemia (ALL)

The only other bispecific antibody besides Removab to have received market approval until the beginning of 2021 is Blincyto, the anti-CD19/anti-CD3 BiTE described above which was approved by the FDA in 2014 for the treatment of patients who have relapsed or are refractory to standard treatment of B-cell acute lymphoblastic leukemia (B-ALL). Approximately 80–90% of adult patients have a remission after chemotherapy, but only 40% achieve a long-term disease-free survival. The presence of minimal residual disease (MRD) after treatment appears to be indicative of a potential relapse. An analysis of 16 clinical trials showed that the absence of MRD was associated with a 10-year survival of 64% compared to only 21% for patients with residual MRD.

In vitro tests with Blincyto demonstrated a very high efficacy for lysing malignant B lymphocytes. Most of them were destroyed in the presence of only picomolar amounts of the bispecific antibody. Interestingly, it was found that Blincyto recruited and activated CD4+ helper T lymphocytes as well as the CD8+ T lymphocytes. It was also demonstrated that one T cell carrying the BiTE could engage in the serial killing of several target cells. However, due to the relatively small size of the BiTEs, they pass unhindered through the kidneys and are quickly removed from the bloodstream. Patients must therefore be continuously infused for several weeks in order to keep the concentration of the drug at a constant level. In order not to restrict the patient's freedom of movement, the drug is administered with the help of a small pump worn on the body.

In a phase III randomized clinical trial (TOWER trial) for the treatment of relapsed/refractory B-ALL, 267 patients received Blincyto and 109 patients received chemotherapy. Induction therapy (the first in a series of therapeutic measures) and consolidation therapy (to consolidate the gains obtained) with Blincyto were administered in a 6-week cycle (4 weeks of treatment and 2 weeks without treatment). Patients received 9 µg per day in the first week followed by 28 µg per day for the next 3 weeks delivered by continuous infusion. Maintenance treatment was given as a 4-week continuous infusion every 12 weeks. Patients with a high tumor load were treated before the trial with dexamethasone to reduce tumor burden and prevent cytokine release syndrome (CRS). Furthermore, all of the patients receiving Blincyto were administered dexamethasone just prior to infusion to prevent infusion reactions.

The overall survival of the relapsed/refractory B-ALL patients receiving Blincyto was 7.7 months versus 4 months for those receiving standard-of-care (SOC) treatment after a follow-up of 11.7 and 11.8 months, respectively. Remission rates for the Blincyto group were 34% CR versus 16% CR for SOC. The frequency of grade 3 or higher adverse events was comparable in the two groups. Blincyto-related neurotoxicity including tremor, dizziness, aphasia, convulsions, and encephalopathy can affect up to half of the patients. However, most of the symptoms are relatively mild and can be managed by administration of dexamethasone without the need to interrupt treatment. Clinical trials to test the efficacy of Blincyto for treating other B-cell malignancies are ongoing.

Recruitment of NK Cells

Most of the bispecific antibodies designed for recruiting NK cells to kill tumor cells by ADCC target CD16A (FcγIIIA), which appears to be the major activation receptor. This receptor is highly homologous (95%) to CD16B (FcγIIIB) on the surface of neutrophils, which, unlike the membrane-spanning CD16A, is anchored to the cell surface through a GPI (glycosylphosphatidylinositol) linker. After neutrophil activation and apoptosis, CD16B is shed by proteolytic cleavage from the cell surface. This results in a constant high level of soluble CD16B in the plasma of healthy individuals due to the daily turnover of apoptotic neutrophils. Antibodies binding

CD16A therefore not only face competition for binding to the Fc receptor on NK cells by the multitude of other serum immunoglobulins but also may be neutralized by soluble CD16B.

To increase the efficacy of NK cell activation using single-chain bispecific antibodies, the biotech firm Affimed in Heidelberg generated an anti-CD16A antibody from a phage display library that is completely specific for CD16A without any binding affinity for the CD16B isoform. Furthermore, the antibody binds to a specific epitope on CD16A distinct from the Fc binding site and displays similar binding properties for both the CD16A alleles 158V/158F described in Chap. 6. Importantly, the binding of the antibody to CD16A showed no significant inhibition by serum IgG. Since Affimed uses antibody formats that are bivalent for CD16A such as the anti-CD30/anti-CD16A TandAb shown in Fig. 9.2, their "ROCK" (redirected optimized cell killing) antibody formats have been engineered to prevent the cross-linking and ensuing fratricide of NK cells, as has been described for some other antibodies.

Other recent constructs for recruiting NK cells include a BiKE (bispecific killer cell engager) antibody, which is similar to a BiTE except that it binds CD16A instead of CD3, and a TriKE (trispecific killer engager), which incorporates an additional scFv-binding domain.

9.8   Risks of Bispecific Antibodies

Under laboratory conditions, bispecific antibodies are much more effective at mediating the lysis of cancer cells than conventional antibodies. Direct comparisons between Rituxan, which has been used very successfully for treating non-Hodgkin lymphoma (see Chap. 6), and Blincyto targeting the same CD19 antigen show a more than 1000-fold higher efficacy for the small bispecific antibody. Similar potencies have been described for other single-chain bispecific antibodies such as TandAbs and DARTs (Fig. 9.1). These high potencies enable cancer cells to be efficiently destroyed, but they also carry the inherent risk of causing severe side effects. After administering Blincyto, for example, the most common adverse events were neurological events, cytokine release syndrome (CRS), cytopenia, elevated liver enzymes, acute pancreatitis, and gastrointestinal disorders. Tumor lysis syndrome was also a major concern since the easily accessible tumor cells in blood cancers can be lysed in a short period of time and their contents released into the bloodstream. This can lead to a metabolic imbalance and impairment of kidney function. Above all, uric acid, the breakdown product of nucleic acids, is often produced in large quantities that can no longer be effectively excreted; it then crystallizes in the kidneys.

The antibody against the tumor antigen could also have an unknown minor affinity for another antigen that would have no consequence with conventional therapeutic antibodies. In the case of a highly potent bispecific antibody, however, the minor affinity might be enough to activate T cells. If the antigen were widespread or expressed on a critical signaling receptor, it could then lead to severe side effects, as in the case of the TeGenero antibody (see Chap. 6). Knowledge of the potential side effects gained in early clinical studies has helped clinicians to devise optimal administration procedures for minimizing the adverse events.

9.9   Targeting Cancers with Chimeric Antigen Receptor (CAR)-T Cells

A method for treating cancer patients using tumor-infiltrating lymphocytes (TILs) harvested from their tumors was described in Chap. 6. The impressive regression of metastatic tumors observed in many of the patients emphasized the potential of autologous T cells for cancer therapy. Modern genetic engineering and antibody engineering techniques have recently facilitated the creation of T cells with defined specificities, improved viability, and robust effector functions. A very detailed account of the history and development of CAR-Ts and bispecific antibodies for recruiting T cells can be found in the review by Strohl and Naso.

9.10   Construction of CARs

The first generation of CARs was produced by fusing an scFv antibody directed against a tumor antigen to the human Fc receptor γ-chain or to the CD3ζ chain (Fig. 9.3). Fcγ and CD3ζ have similar sequences comprising a short extracellular domain, a transmembrane domain, and the immunoreceptor tyrosine-based activation motif (ITAM; see Chap. 2). These first constructs, however, were not very successful and lacked the ability to proliferate and persist in the circulation.

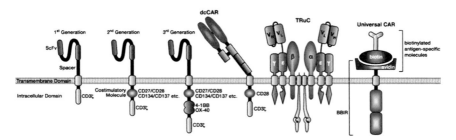

Fig. 9.3 Evolving design of chimeric antigen receptor T cells (CAR-Ts). (1) Three generations of CAR design starting with scFv fused to a CD3ζ chain and then with the addition of costimulation domains; (2) dual chain CAR (dcCAR) where one half of a mAb is fused to receptor domains; (3) T-cell receptor fusion construct (TRuC) where an scFv is fused to CD3ε of the T-cell receptor; (4) universal CAR utilizing the biotin-avidin system (BBIR: biotin-binding immune receptor). Other alternative universal systems include T cells transduced with CD16 CARs which bind the Fc domain of any IgG1 mAb. (From Hughes-Parry HE, Cross R S, Jenkins MR (2019) Int. J. Mol. Sci. 2020, 21, 204; doi:https://doi.org/10.3390/ijms21010204. Permission for use according to creative commons license (http://creativecommons.org/licenses/by/4.0/))

One reason for their failure was thought to be the lack of a costimulatory signal. A second generation of CAR-T cells was therefore made by adding a cytoplasmic signaling domain from a costimulatory molecule such as CD28, 4-1BB (CD137), or OX40 (CD134). These constructs resulted in an increased production of activating cytokines such as IL-2 and IFN-γ and increased proliferation, but T-cell activation was still not optimal. A third generation of CARs was therefore designed incorporating intracellular signaling domains from CD28 plus those of OX40 or 4-1BB, resulting in better proliferation, persistence in the circulation, and killing potential. Further improvements in CAR activity were achieved by optimizing the length and structure of the extracellular spacer to achieve a flexible hinge region using suitable regions from IgG-Fc or CD8 (Fig. 9.3).

The two CAR-T cells approved for clinical use by the FDA at the time of writing, Kymriah and Yescarta, are second-generation products containing a costimulatory sequence fused to CD3ζ for intracellular signaling.

9.11   Kymriah for Treating B-ALL: The First Gene Therapy to Be Approved by the FDA

The CAR-T cell Kymriah (tisagenlecleucel) was approved by the FDA in 2017 for the treatment of patients up to 25 years of age with B-cell precursor acute lymphoblastic leukemia (ALL) that is refractory or has relapsed at least twice. It expresses a CAR comprising an anti-CD19 single-chain antibody (scFv) on the cell surface fused via a transmembrane domain to cytoplasmic signaling domains of costimulatory receptor 4-1BB (CD137) and CD3ζ of the T-cell receptor complex.

The pivotal clinical trial leading to approval was a global, multicenter, single-arm phase II study (the ELIANA trial). Treatment consisted of administering fludarabine and cyclophosphamide followed 2–14 days later by a single dose of Kymriah. Autologous peripheral blood mononuclear cells were collected locally by leukapheresis from enrolled patients and shipped to a manufacturing facility where they were enriched for T cells. After activation with anti-CD3/CD28 antibody-coated beads, the T cells were transduced with a lentiviral vector encoding the anti-CD19 CAR, expanded ex vivo, and formulated into a cryopreserved product. The maximal number of cells in a single dose was 2.5×10^8. The complete response (CR) rate was 63%, and all CRs had minimal residual disease (MRD) <0.01%. There were some serious cytotoxicities with 79% of the patients suffering from cytokine release syndrome (CRS) and 65% from neurologic side effects, many requiring intensive care treatment. CRS in these patients is typically characterized by very high levels of the inflammatory cytokine IL6. Patients are therefore very often treated with RoActemra (tocilizumab), an anti-IL6 antibody, and, if this is not sufficient, by the administration of steroids. The very impressive results achieved in patients with chemotherapy-refractory B-ALL were considered to be sufficiently compelling evidence of clinical benefit to justify a regular rather than an accelerated approval. In 2018 Kymriah was also approved for the treatment of refractory or relapsed diffuse large B-cell lymphoma.

One major drawback is the price. The cost of one treatment for patients with B-ALL is about $475,000.

9.12   Yescarta for Treating Diffuse Large B-Cell Lymphoma (DLBCL)

The FDA granted regular approval for the CAR-T cell Yescarta (axicabtagene ciloleucel) in 2017 for the treatment of adult patients with relapsed or refractory DLBCL after two or more lines of systemic therapy. Yescarta comprises an extracellular anti-CD19 scFv fused via a transmembrane domain to the signaling domains of the costimulatory receptor CD28 (instead of 4-1BB as in Kymriah) and CD3ζ. Its preparation and administration were very similar to the protocol for Kymriah. The objective response rate was 72% with a CR rate of 51%. Serious adverse reactions occurred in 52% of the patients. Ninety-four percent of the patients experienced cytokine release syndrome and 74% neurologic toxicities. Following the results of a parallel clinical trial, Yescarta was also approved in 2017 for the treatment of primary mediastinal large B-cell lymphoma (PMBCL). On the downside, one treatment for a patient with DLBCL costs about $373,000.

The large number of patients with serious side effects led to the implementation of a risk evaluation and mitigation strategy. In the case of Kymriah and Yescarta, the CD19 target is expressed at a high level on most types of B lymphocyte. This may have resulted in an overactivation that may not occur with more selective targeting and less abundant target molecules. Ongoing research into the factors driving CRS may also open up new approaches for controlling CRS as more is learned about the mechanisms involved.

9.13   Novel Approaches to Optimize CAR-T Therapy

Dual Chain CAR (dcCAR) and Antibody Mimetics

Instead of using a single-chain antibody to target tumor cells, the dcCAR approach uses the natural form of an antibody by expressing the heavy and light chains simultaneously (Fig. 9.3). The heavy chain is fused to the signaling domains and is linked to the light chain with disulfide bonds. One of the benefits of this approach is that all mAbs can readily be expressed in this format, they are more stable than scFvs, and evidence has been provided that they may function better and result in lower levels of cytokine secretion. More data, however, is needed to support these claims.

T-Cell Receptor Fusion Constructs (TRuCs)

TRuCs comprise an scFv fused to the T-cell receptor subunit CD3ε (Fig. 9.3). They are a functional component of the TCR complex which employ the full signaling machinery of the TCR complex independent of HLA as opposed to CARs that use the limited signaling capacity of an isolated CD3ζ cytoplasmic tail. TRuCs targeting CD19 were just as potent as second-generation CAR-T cells despite the absence of an extra costimulatory domain, and they appear to cause significantly lower amounts of cytokine release.

Universal Immune Receptors (UIRs)

Tumor cells can evade CAR-T cells by downregulating the expression of tumor-associated antigens. It would therefore be useful to have a universal docking mechanism for creating CAR-T cells able to target any desired antigen. This can be achieved by docking pairs such as avidin-biotin shown in Fig. 9.3. Any biotinylated antibody can be captured by avidin coupled to the intracellular signaling domains. If the avidin proves to be unacceptably immunogenic, there are many alternative universal linking systems such as leucine zippers or the fusion of the CD16A (FcγRIIIA) high-affinity variant V158 to the CAR-T cell intracellular signaling domains. This latter construct binds strongly to the antibody Fc domain, thus providing an effective universal chimeric receptor for targeting tumor cells with any IgG antibody. The UIRs would be particularly useful for manufacturing relatively inexpensive off-the-shelf CAR-T cells derived from allogenic donors (see below).

Prevention of T-Cell Exhaustion and Immunosuppression

A major problem in the treatment of solid tumors is T-cell exhaustion resulting from chronic stimulation. This commonly occurs in the immunosuppressive tumor microenvironment. Exhausted T cells often overexpress inhibitory markers such as PD-1, LAG-3, and TIM-3 and are impaired in their ability to release pro-inflammatory cytokines such as IFNγ and TNFα. CAR-T cells have therefore been engineered to secrete and deliver PD-1, CTLA-4, or PD-L1 antibodies or stimulatory cytokines at the tumor site. Another interesting approach is to generate CAR-T cells that secrete a bispecific antibody such as a BiTE binding to the same or a different tumor antigen with one of its binding sites and to the CD3 complex of a TCR with the other binding site. This could help to stimulate bystander tumor infiltrating T lymphocytes as well as providing pro-inflammatory cytokines to enhance CAR-T cell cytotoxic activity.

Synthesis of Orthogonal Cytokines and Receptors

T cells have been engineered to express an orthogonal mutant IL-2 receptor (ortho-IL-2R) that can only be activated by an orthogonal mutant IL-2 (ortho-IL-2). This facilitates the administration of ortho-IL-2 for stimulating transduced cancer-specific T cells without the risk of activating normal T cells. In a preclinical murine model system, the addition of high doses of ortho-IL-2 to a mixture of adoptively transferred wild-type T cells and ortho-IL-2R T cells resulted in the expansion of only the ortho-IL-2R T cells, thus facilitating improved tumor cell killing without a systemic IL-2 toxicity.

Deletion of Regnase-1

Activated T cells often become less functional in the tumor microenvironment. The ribonuclease regnase-1 has been identified as a major regulator of cytotoxic T-cell function. Gene-modified CD8+ T cells that do not express regnase-1 persist longer in tumors, have an enhanced metabolism, and express more effector molecules. They also increase the survival times of tumor-bearing mice. A mRNA encoding the transcription factor BATF was identified as the major target of regnase-1, since deletion of BATF abolished the antitumor activity of regnase-1-deleted T cells.

Priming CAR-T Cells by Antigen-Presenting Cells (APCs)

Two promising strategies involving APCs have been developed to overcome ineffi-cient CAR-T cell stimulation in vivo for the treatment of solid tumors.

Bispecific CARs targeting APCs and tumors. To stimulate proliferation and prime CAR-T cells for tumor cell killing, an amphiphile ligand carrying FITC (fluorescein isothiocyanate) was designed by a group of scientists at the MIT headed by Darrell Irvine that after injection into mice trafficked to the lymph nodes and decorated the cell membrane of antigen-presenting cells (APCs) with the ligand (see Ma et al.). CAR-T cells carrying bispecific antibodies binding to both the FITC antigen and to tumor antigens were stimulated to proliferate after being primed by binding to the APCs in the native lymph node microenvironment. The expanded CAR-T cells displayed enhanced antitumor efficacy in immunocompe-tent mouse tumor models.

Vaccine boosting of CAR-T cell efficacy. A nanoparticulate RNA vaccine was designed for the delivery of tumor-associated antigens into lymphoid compart-ments. The presentation of the natively folded target on resident antigen-presenting cells promoted the selective expansion of CAR-T cells that targeted the same tumor antigen. This resulted in the improved engraftment of the CAR-T cells and the regression of large tumors in difficult-to-treat mouse models using only subthera-peutic CAR-T cell doses.

9.14   Allogenic CARs

The production of individual autologous CAR-T cells is an expensive process. To decrease the financial burden, considerable research has been invested in the design of allogenic off-the-shelf products, and an increasing number are entering clinical trials. A major problem using allogenic CAR-T cells is that they are usually not histocompatible and may be rejected by the patient's immune system or cause graft versus host disease (GVHD). In recent generations of allogenic CAR-T cells, the genes coding for HLA class I proteins have been deleted to reduce the risk of rejection. GVHD can also be avoided by deleting genes such as TRAC (coding for TCR-α) to prevent the formation of a TCR. However, cells without classical HLA class I are targets for cytotoxic NK cells due to the absence of the HLA ligand for the inhibitory KIR receptor. One approach to solve this potential problem has been to express nonclassical HLA class molecules such as HLA-E or HLA-G, which have been shown to protect cells from lysis by NK cells and are much less immunogenic than classical HLA.

9.15   NK CARs and Macrophage CARs

Another approach to avoid GVHD is to use NK cells, since they have no TCR. However, these cells are eventually rejected by the immune system, thus limiting their ability to expand and persist, which are important factors for achieving good responses and long-term remissions. Alternative CAR cells that are being investigated for allogenic products are NKT cells, which share characteristics of both NK and T cells, gamma/delta (γ/δ) T cells (see Chap. 2), and even macrophages.

Macrophages are particularly interesting as potential CAR cells because of their capacity to penetrate tumors, where M2 macrophages often represent a substantial part of the tumor mass. Using a chimeric adenoviral vector, scientists at the University of Pennsylvania School of Medicine genetically engineered human macrophages with CARs to direct their phagocytic activity against tumors. This manipulation resulted in CAR macrophages with a sustained pro-inflammatory M1 phenotype which were able to convert bystander M2 macrophages to M1 and which were resistant to the effects of immunosuppressive cytokines. In in vitro experiments and mouse models, they proved to be very effective at reducing tumor burden.

9.16   T Cells Transduced with a Cancer-Specific TCR

As described in Chaps. 2 and 3, a human T-cell clone has been isolated that was shown by CRISPR-Cas9 screening of the genome to bind a cancer-specific ligand via the monomorphic MHC class I-related protein, MR1. When the TCR of this clone was transduced into T cells from the PBMCs of stage IV melanoma patients, it redirected them to kill autologous and non-autologous melanoma cells but not healthy cells. Since the TCR recognizes diverse cancer cell types, including primary cancer cells, it opens up the possibility of developing a universal T-cell-mediated cancer immunotherapy as an alternative to the CAR-Ts described above.

9.17   Safety Switches

One of the major risks of very efficacious autologous CAR cell products and, more recently, non-immunogenic allogeneic products is the possibility of an uncontrolled expansion and subsequent excessive stimulation of the immune system. Many CAR cell products have therefore been designed to incorporate a safety switch.

A widely used "kill switch" is CaspaCIDE®, which couples an inducible caspase-9 (iCasp9) with a small molecule inducer known as AP1903. After administration of AP1903, the expression of caspase-9 leads to a rapid destruction of the CAR cells. Another popular method to kill CAR cells is to display the epitope of an approved antibody capable of inducing cell lysis by ADCC. For example, a peptide comprising the epitope recognized by the approved anti-EGFR antibody Erbitux has been fused with a mammalian leader sequence for expression on the cell surface. Administration of Erbitux results in the elimination of cells expressing the EGFR marker. This tag is also useful for sorting and tracking the CAR-T cells. Similarly, a peptide comprising the epitope of the anti-CD20 antibody Rituxan has been incorporated into the hinge region of CARs in some allogeneic cells to facilitate their elimination by ADCC.

Selected Literature

Baeuerle PA, Ding J, Patel E, et al. Synthetic TRuC receptors engaging the complete T cell receptor for potent anti-tumor response. Nat Commun. 2019;10(1):2087. https://doi.org/10.1038/s41467-019-10097-0.

Brinkmann U, Kontermann RE. The making of bispecific antibodies. MAbs. 2017;9(2):182–212. https://doi.org/10.1080/19420862.2016.1268307.

Burt R, Warcel D, Fielding AK. Blinatumomab, a bispecific B-cell and T-cell engaging antibody, in the treatment of B-cell malignancies. Hum Vaccin Immunother. 2019;15(3):594–602. https://doi.org/10.1080/21645515.2018.1540828.

Chiu ML, Goulet DR, Teplyakov A, Gilliland GL. Antibody structure and function: the basis for engineering therapeutics. Antibodies. 2019;8(4):55. https://doi.org/10.3390/antib8040055.

Crowther MD, Dolton G, Legut M, et al. Genome-wide CRISPR-Cas9 screening reveals ubiquitous T cell cancer targeting via the monomorphic MHC class I-related protein MR1 [published correction appears in Nat Immunol. 2020 Mar 2]. Nat Immunol. 2020;21(2):178–85. https://doi.org/10.1038/s41590-019-0578-8.

Ellwanger K, Reusch U, Fucek I, et al. Redirected optimized cell killing (ROCK®): a highly versatile multispecific fit-for-purpose antibody platform for engaging innate immunity. MAbs. 2019;11(5):899–918. https://doi.org/10.1080/19420862.2019.1616506.

Felices M, Lenvik TR, Davis ZB, et al. Generation of BiKEs and TriKEs to improve NK cell-mediated targeting of tumor cells. Methods Mol Biol. 2016;1441:333–46. https://doi.org/10.1007/978-1-4939-3684-7_28.

Gong S, Ren F, Wu D, et al. Fabs-in-tandem immunoglobulin is a novel and versatile bispecific design for engaging multiple therapeutic targets. MAbs. 2017;9(7):1118–28. https://doi.org/10.1080/19420862.2017.1345401.

Haas C, Krinner E, Brischwein K, et al. Mode of cytotoxic action of T cell-engaging BiTE antibody MT110. Immunobiology. 2009;214:441–53.

Hughes-Parry HE, Cross RS, Jenkins MR. The evolving protein engineering in the design of chimeric antigen receptor T cells. Int J Mol Sci. 2019;21(1):204. https://doi.org/10.3390/ijms21010204.

Kantarjian H, Stein A, Gökbuget N, et al. Blinatumomab versus chemotherapy for advanced acute lymphoblastic leukemia. N Engl J Med. 2017;376(9):836–47. https://doi.org/10.1056/NEJMoa1609783.

Klichinsky M, Ruella M, Shestova O, et al. Human chimeric antigen receptor macrophages for cancer immunotherapy. Nat Biotechnol. 2020;38:947–53. https://doi.org/10.1038/s41587-020-0462-y.

Kontermann R, Brinkmann U. Bispecific antibodies. Drug Discov Today. 2015;20:838–47. https://doi.org/10.1016/j.drudis.2015.02.008.

Ma L, Dichwalkar T, Chang JYH, et al. Enhanced CAR-T cell activity against solid tumors by vaccine boosting through the chimeric receptor. Science. 2019;365(6449):162–8. https://doi.org/10.1126/science.aav8692.

Minetto P, Guolo F, Pesce S, et al. Harnessing NK cells for cancer treatment. Front Immunol. 2019;10:2836. https://doi.org/10.3389/fimmu.2019.02836.

Reinhard K, Rengstl B, Oehm P, et al. An RNA vaccine drives expansion and efficacy of claudin-CAR-T cells against solid tumors. Science. 2020;367(6476):446–53. https://doi.org/10.1126/science.aay5967.

Reusch U, Duell J, Ellwanger K, et al. A tetravalent bispecific TandAb (CD19/CD3), AFM11, efficiently recruits T cells for the potent lysis of CD19(+) tumor cells. MAbs. 2015;7(3):584–604. https://doi.org/10.1080/19420862.2015.1029216.

Ross SL, Sherman M, McElroy PL, et al. Bispecific T cell engager (BiTE®) antibody constructs can mediate bystander tumor cell killing. PLoS One. 2017;12(8):e0183390. https://doi.org/10.1371/journal.pone.0183390.

Sacchetti B, Botticelli A, Pierelli L, et al. CAR-T with license to kill solid tumors in search of a winning strategy. Int J Mol Sci. 2019;20:1903. https://doi.org/10.3390/ijms20081903.

Sedykh SE, Prinz VV, Buneva VN, Nevinsky GA. Bispecific antibodies: design, therapy, perspectives. Drug Des Dev Ther. 2018;12:195–208. https://doi.org/10.2147/DDDT.S151282.

Shim H. Bispecific antibodies and antibody-drug conjugates for cancer therapy: technological considerations. Biomol Ther. 2020;10(3):360. https://doi.org/10.3390/biom10030360.

Sockolosky JT, Trotta E, Parisi G, et al. Selective targeting of engineered T cells using orthogonal IL-2 cytokine-receptor complexes. Science. 2018;359(6379):1037–42. https://doi.org/10.1126/science.aar3246.

Spiess C, Zhai Q, Carter PJ. Alternative molecular formats and therapeutic applications for bispecific antibodies. Mol Immunol. 2015;67:95–106. https://doi.org/10.1016/j.molimm.2015.01.003.

Strohl WR, Naso M. Bispecific T-cell redirection versus chimeric antigen receptor (CAR)-T cells as approaches to kill cancer cells. Antibodies. 2019;8(3):41. https://doi.org/10.3390/antib8030041.

Suurs FV, Lub-de Hooge MN, de Vries EGE, de Groot DJA. A review of bispecific antibodies and antibody constructs in oncology and clinical challenges. Pharmacol Ther. 2019;201:103–19. https://doi.org/10.1016/j.pharmthera.2019.04.006.

Wang Q, Chen Y, Park J, et al. Design and production of bispecific antibodies. Antibodies. 2019;8(3):43. https://doi.org/10.3390/antib8030043.

Wei J, Long L, Zheng W, et al. Targeting regnase-1 programs long-lived effector T cells for cancer therapy. Nature. 2019;576(7787):471–6. https://doi.org/10.1038/s41586-019-1821-z.

Xie G, Dong H, Liang Y, Ham JD, Rizwan R, Chen J. CAR-NK cells: a promising cellular immunotherapy for cancer. EBioMedicine. 2020;102975:59. https://doi.org/10.1016/j.ebiom.2020.102975.

Yasunaga M. Antibody therapeutics and immunoregulation in cancer and autoimmune disease. Semin Cancer Biol. 2020;64:1–12. https://doi.org/10.1016/j.semcancer.2019.06.001.

Zah E, Lin MY, Silva-Benedict A, Jensen MC, Chen YY. T cells expressing CD19/CD20 bispecific chimeric antigen receptors prevent antigen escape by malignant B cells. Cancer Immunol Res. 2016;4(6):498–508. https://doi.org/10.1158/2326-6066.CIR-15-0231.

Zhao L, Cao YJ. Engineered T cell therapy for cancer in the clinic. Front Immunol. 2019;10:2250. https://doi.org/10.3389/fimmu.2019.02250.

Cancer Incidence: Market for Therapeutic Antibodies

10

Abstract

Approximately 450 per 100,000 people are newly diagnosed with cancer each year in the United States, and about 160 per 100,000 people die of cancer. The risk of US citizens getting cancer at some point in their lives is 40%, and about 21% of men and 18% of women risk dying of cancer. Four types of cancer, lung, colorectal, breast, and prostate, account for a fourth of all cancer deaths. In China, about 36% of deaths were due to stomach, liver, and esophagus cancer with relatively poor prognoses. In the United States and the United Kingdom, however, these cancers only accounted for ≤5% of the mortalities. The estimated national expenditures for cancer care in the United States in 2018 were $150.8 billion, which could rise significantly due to the increasing use of novel therapeutic antibodies. The antibody Keytruda, for example, directed against the checkpoint inhibitor PD-1, is soon expected to overtake Humira as the top-selling biological drug. The median price of mAbs for 1 year of treatment in the United States in the area of oncology/hematology in 2019 was about $143,000. To facilitate decisions regarding reimbursement, some countries have established cost-effectiveness thresholds.

10.1 Introduction

The acquisition of the biotech firm Genentech, which developed Rituxan/MabThera (rituximab) together with Biogen Idec, enabled Roche to establish an early dominant position in the market for treating cancer with therapeutic antibodies. In order not to be left behind, other large pharmaceutical companies invested heavily in the acquisition of key antibody technologies and antibody biotech firms. An overview of cancer incidence, cancer mortalities, the market for therapeutic antibodies, the process for obtaining market approval of antibody product candidates, and other related topics are described below.

10.2   Market for Treating Cancer with Antibodies

In an annual report to the nation (United States) on the status of cancer (part II) in 2020 by Jane Henley and colleagues, the most common causes of cancer death among females were lung, breast, and colorectal cancers. Among males, the three most common were lung, prostate, and colorectal cancers. Twenty-four percent of all cancer deaths were from lung cancers, 9% from colorectal cancers, 7% from breast cancers, and 5% from prostate cancers. Together, these four cancers accounted for almost half of deaths due to cancer (Fig. 10.1). Pancreatic cancer (7%) was the fourth most common cause of cancer death among both females and males, followed by liver and intrahepatic bile duct cancer, leukemia, and non-Hodgkin lymphoma. Deaths due to other types of cancer accounted individually for less than 3% of cancer deaths.

Fig. 10.1   Cancer deaths for both sexes, all ages, and ethnicities combined—United States, 2017. (From Henley et al. Cancer 2020; 126:2250–2266 by permission of John Wiley and Sons)

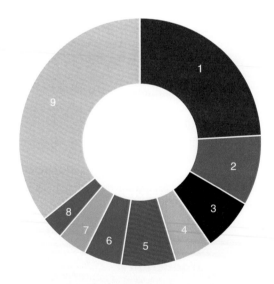

■ 1. LUNG AND BRONCHUS	(24%)
■ 2. COLON AND RECTUM	(9%)
■ 3. FEMALE BREAST	(7%)
▨ 4. PROSTATE	(5%)
■ 5. PANCREAS	(7%)
■ 6. LIVER AND INTRAHEPATIC BILE DUCT	(5%)
▨ 7. LEUKEMIAS	(4%)
■ 8. NON-HODGKIN LYMPHOMA	(3%)
▨ 9. ALL OTHER CANCERS	(35%)

10.3   Cancer Mortality in United States

Approximately 600,000 people died from cancer in 2017 in the United States, and about three times that number were newly diagnosed with cancer representing an incidence of 448 per 100,000 people. The yearly cancer mortality rate was higher among men than women; 189 per 100,000 for men and 136 per 100,000 for women. Based on race/ethnicity and sex, cancer mortality is highest in African American men (233 per 100,000) and lowest in Asian/Pacific Islander women (86 per 100,000). The estimated national expenditures for cancer care in the United States in 2018 were $150.8 billion.

10.4   Comparison of Mortality Rates Between China and the United States/United Kingdom

It is interesting to compare the above statistics for the United States with those of China, which represents a country in transition from a developing country to a developed country. Feng and colleagues in "Cancer Communications" (2019) reported that the age-standardized cancer incidence in China in 2018 was about 200/100,000, which is comparable to the overall worldwide incidence but lower than in the United Kingdom (319/100,000) or the United States (352/100,000). However, China had a higher mortality rate of about 130/100,000 compared to 103/100,000 for the United Kingdom and 91/100,000 for the United States, which might reflect a different pattern of cancers, lower early detection rates, or differences in treatment. These figures differ from the absolute values for the United States shown above because they have been age-standardized in order to allow for the proportion of people in corresponding age groups. A major difference in the pattern of cancer-related deaths in China and the United States/United Kingdom was that 36.4% of deaths in China were due to digestive tract cancers (stomach 13.6%, liver 12.9%, esophagus cancer 9.9%) with relatively poor prognoses. In the United States, the age-standardized mortality for these cancers totaled 13.8% (stomach 3.1%, liver 6.6%, esophagus 3.9%), similar to the situation in the United Kingdom. The five most common cancer mortalities in China are lung (24%), stomach (13%), liver (13%) esophagus (10%), and colorectal (8%). Most of the mortalities due to cancer of the esophagus occurred in the male population.

10.5   Risk of Developing Cancer

An investigation published in Nature in 2016 by Song Wu and colleagues concluded that intrinsic factors relating to random DNA mutations account for less than 10–30% of cancer development, with at least 70% being due to extrinsic risk factors. Although this data has been contested by other research scientists, it is generally agreed that the risk of getting cancer is significantly increased by lifestyle and environmental factors such as tobacco, alcohol, sunbathing, viral infections, carcinogens, and diet. The likelihood of developing cancer in the course of a lifetime for US citizens was statistically assessed by the National Cancer Institute in 2020 for the period 2014–2016 (Table 10.1). According to these data, 40.1% of men and 38.7% of women risk developing cancer, and 21.3% of men and 18.4% of women have a risk of dying from cancer.

The chances of recovery from cancer depend largely on individual factors. However, for each type of cancer, there is a general prognosis about the likelihood that a patient can be cured. The 5-year survival rate, for example, is the percentage of people with a specific cancer who are still alive 5 years after diagnosis. Current evidence indicates that the likelihood of a cure after 5 years with no symptoms is relatively high.

An extensive study on the survival rate of US citizens with cancer for the period 1975–2016 was carried out in the SEER program ("Surveillance, Epidemiology, and End Results") of the National Cancer Institute (Table 10.2). Significant

Table 10.1 Lifetime probability of developing and dying from cancer in United States, 2014–2016

	Males				Females			
	Developing		Dying		Developing		Dying	
	1 in…	%	1 in…	%	1 in…	%	1 in…	%
All sites[a]	2	40.1	5	21.3	3	38.7	5	18.4
Prostate	9	11.6	41	2.4	–	–	–	–
Lung and bronchus	15	6.7	18	5.5	17	6.0	22	4.5
Colorectal	23	4.4	55	1.8	25	4.1	60	1.7
Urinary bladder[b]	26	3.9	107	0.9	85	1.2	289	0.3
Melanoma of skin[c]	28	3.6	210	0.5	41	2.5	425	0.2
Non-Hodgkin lymphoma	41	2.4	124	0.8	52	1.9	157	0.6
Kidney and renal pelvis	46	2.2	166	0.6	82	1.2	306	0.3
Leukemia	54	1.9	104	1.0	77	1.3	146	0.7
Pancreas	60	1.7	72	1.4	62	1.6	74	1.4
Oral cavity and pharynx	60	1.7	238	0.4	141	0.7	538	0.2
Liver and intrahepatic bile duct	69	1.4	98	1.0	162	0.6	186	0.5
Stomach	94	1.1	224	0.4	151	0.7	332	0.3
Myeloma	107	0.9	212	0.5	141	0.7	263	0.4
Esophagus	126	0.8	132	0.8	415	0.2	502	0.2
Brain and ONS	145	0.7	188	0.5	183	0.5	238	0.4
Thyroid	144	0.7	1724	0.1	52	1.9	1399	0.1
Larynx	189	0.5	529	0.2	786	0.1	2143	< 0.1
Testis	247	0.4	5015	<0.1	–	–	–	–
Hodgkin lymphoma	418	0.2	2588	<0.1	510	0.2	3555	<0.1
Breast	750	0.1	3217	<0.1	8	12.8	39	2.6
Ovary	–	–	–	–	80	1.3	114	0.9
Uterine corpus	–	–	–	–	33	3.1	159	0.6
Uterine cervix	–	–	–	–	159	0.6	453	0.2

Software: DevCan—Probability of developing or dying of cancer software, version 6.7.7, National Cancer Institute, 2019

[a]All sites excludes basal cell and squamous cell skin cancers and in situ cancers except urinary bladder

[b]Includes invasive and in situ cancer cases

[c]Statistics are for non-Hispanic whites

Table 10.2   5-year relative survival rates in the United States by stage at diagnosis

	All	All	Local	Regional	Distant
	1987–1989	2009–2015	2009–2015	2009–2015	2009–2015
Prostate	83	98	>99	>99	31
Breast (female)	84	90	99	86	27
Lung and bronchus	13	19	57	31	5
Colorectal	60	65	90	71	14
Urinary bladder	79	77[a]	70	36	5
Melanoma of skin	88	92	99	65	25
Kidney and renal pelvis	57	75	93	70	12
Pancreas	4	9	37	12	3
Oral cavity and pharynx	54	65	84	66	39
Liver and intrahepatic bile duct	5	18	33	11	2
Stomach	20	32	69	31	5
Testis	95	95	99	96	73
Ovary	38	48	92	75	29
Thyroid	94	98	>99	98	56
Esophagus	9	19	47	25	5
Non-Hodgkin lymphoma	51	75			
Myeloma	27	54			
Leukemia	43	66			

Local: Malignant cancer confined to organ of origin. **Regional**: Malignant cancer that has extended into neighboring organs or tissues and/or involves regional lymph nodes. **Distant**: Malignant cancer that has spread to distant organs, tissues, or lymph nodes
Source: Noone AM, Howlader N, Krapcho et al. (eds). SEER Cancer Statistics Review, 1975–2016, National Cancer Institute. Bethesda, MD. https://seer.cancer.gov/csr/1975_2016/, based on November 2018 SEER data submission, posted to the SEER web site, April 2019
[a]Rate for in situ cases is 95%

improvements in this time period due to earlier diagnoses and/or improvements in cancer treatment were observed for nearly all types of cancer, particularly prostate, breast, colon, rectum, and leukemia. The survival rate for patients with cancer of the pancreas and of the lungs and bronchi also improved but remained at a relatively low level. On the whole, figures released in March 2020 in the "Annual Report to the Nation" showed that cancer death rates had decreased by 1.8% per year for men and 1.4% per year for women during 2001–2017.

10.6   Cancer Therapies

The most common treatments for cancer are surgical removal, radiation, and chemotherapy. Surgery and radiation are particularly effective in patients with localized cancers. However, a systemic drug treatment is needed for tumors that have already spread due to the formation of metastases or that cannot be removed by surgery.

Chemotherapy often involves the administration of a combination of different drugs that inhibit the growth or division of cancer cells, the goal being to kill as many cancer cells as possible in the sensitive phase of cell division (mitosis). Several cycles of treatment are therefore necessary, since only a small fraction of the cells undergo mitosis at a given time. Unfortunately, fast-growing cells in the body such as cells of the digestive tract, ovaries, and hair roots are also affected. This leads to side effects such as hair loss, nausea, vomiting, loss of appetite, fever, inflammation of the mucous membranes, and diarrhea. Moreover, since the generation of new blood cells is also impaired, the immune system is less effective at fighting infections.

The development of therapies that destroy cancer cells without affecting the whole body is a major goal of cancer research (Paul Ehrlich's "Magic Bullets"; see Chap. 7). To find the vulnerable Achilles heel of tumor cells, considerable resources have been invested into basic research on the differences between cancer cells and normal cells. For example, the so-called Philadelphia chromosome was found in over 90% of patients with chronic myeloid leukemia (CML). This is a shortened chromosome 22, which has exchanged genetic material with chromosome 9 through a reciprocal translocation, whereby the tyrosine-protein kinase ABL gene becomes fused to the BCR gene ("breakpoint cluster region" gene). As a BCR-ABL fusion protein, the kinase activity of ABL is no longer regulated by cytokines and is constitutively active. This results in an uncontrolled increase in white blood cells that play a crucial role in the development of CML. A search for substances that effectively inhibit ABL tyrosine kinase resulted in the discovery of the inhibitor Gleevec® (imatinib mesylate) with which many patients have been cured.

Another development towards cancer-specific therapy was the production of antibodies directed against tumor-associated antigens (TAAs). This branch of the pharmaceutical industry experienced an unprecedented growth in the last 20 years. The profits from therapeutic antibodies, for example, now represent a major source of revenue for several large pharmaceutical firms such as Roche.

10.7   Acquisition of Genentech by Roche

On a Friday evening in 1973 after a busy week, Herbert Boyer showed his wife pictures of bands on a gel that he had taken with a Polaroid camera. He was euphoric; he and Stanley Cohen had succeeded in recombining DNA from different organisms and reproducing it in bacteria. Boyer couldn't stop looking at the picture of the bands until early in the morning. He was very moved, and his eyes welled up with tears as he had a cloudy vision of what was to come. However, although many scientists were very impressed by this work at the time, further developments to manufacture genetic engineering products seemed to be far away.

That view was not shared by Robert Swanson, 29, who had both a bachelor's degree in chemistry and a master's in management. Having a somewhat insecure position in an investment company, he was looking for a suitable opportunity to start a biotechnology company. Since he was particularly fascinated by the possibilities of recombinant DNA technology, he sought a conversation with Herbert Boyer, who reluctantly granted him an interview for a few minutes. After a conversation that then lasted several hours, the idea to found Genentech was born.

In the early years of its existence after being founded in 1976, Genentech developed a number of breakthrough biological products, including human insulin and human growth hormone that resulted in a meteoric rise to become a major biotechnological company. Its products attracted the attention of major pharmaceutical companies, and Roche in Basel acquired a major stake in Genentech's shares in 1990. Eighteen years later, in 2009, Roche acquired the remaining shares for the enormous sum of approximately $47 billion. This high-risk business venture paid off in full for Roche; only 4 years later, it had recuperated most of the money spent on the acquisition and is now one of the leading companies in the field of therapeutic antibodies for treating cancer. Although the revenues of its three leading antibody products Herceptin, Avastin, and Rituxan are gradually dwindling due to the emergence of copycat biosimilars, it has a large number of additional antibodies for treating cancer in the pipeline. At the time of writing, Roche was the third largest pharmaceutical company after Johnson & Johnson and Pfizer with total revenues per year of approximately $50bn. Interestingly, antibodies for cancer therapy that target checkpoint inhibitors now earn more revenues than antibodies targeting tumor antigens or tumor vasculature (Table 10.3). Indeed, the anti-PD-1 mAb Keytruda has been forecasted to topple Humira from its long-standing bestseller position in the next few years.

The rapid success of Rituxan (rituximab) took many pharmaceutical companies by surprise. Hardly any of them had made a significant contribution to the development of antibody technology and had overlooked an important development in the

Table 10.3 Top ten pharmaceutical products by global sales in 2019

	Pharmaceutical product (Ab = antibody)	Main indication	Company	Revenue $bn
1	Humira (adalimumab) Human anti-TNF Ab	Rheumatoid arthritis	AbbVie	~19.7
2	Keytruda (pembrolizumab) Humanized anti-PD-1	11 types of cancer	Merck & Co.	~11.1
3	Revlimid (lenalidomide)	Multiple myeloma	Bristol Myers Squibb (Celgene)	~11.1
4	Opdivo (nivolumab) Human anti-PD-1	10 types of cancer	Bristol Myers Squibb	~8.1
5	Eylea (aflibercept) Anti-VDGFR1&2 fusion mAb	Wet macular degeneration	Regeneron, Bayer	~8.0
6	Eliquis (apixaban)	Anticoagulant	Bristol Myers Squibb, Pfizer	~7.9
7	Enbrel (etanercept) TNF receptor fusion mAb	Rheumatoid arthritis	Amgen	~7.2
8	Avastin (bevacizumab) humanized anti-VEGF-A mAb	Various cancers	Roche	~7.1
9	Stelara (ustekinumab) human mAb against p40 (IL12, IL23)	Psoriasis	Johnson & Johnson	~6.6
10	Rituxan (US)/MabThera (EU) chimeric anti-CD20 mAb	Non-Hodgkin lymphoma, CLL, RA	Roche, Johnson & Johnson	~6.5

Data from FiercePharma: https://www.fiercepharma.com/special-report/top-20-drugs-by-global-sales-2019

field of biopharmaceuticals. Taking Roche as an example, several of the large pharmaceutical companies managed to build up a biopharmaceutical division with a focus on antibodies through takeovers or mergers. Two outstanding examples are the merger of Schering-Plough with Merck in 2009 and the acquisition of Wyeth by Pfizer for $68 billion in 2009.

10.8   Acquisition of Antibody Technologies

Virtually all biotech companies with patented antibody production technologies that do not infringe the patent rights of other companies have been taken over by large firms. Amgen, for example, bought Abgenix for $2.2 billion, and Bristol-Meyers Squibb paid a similar price to acquire Medarex. Table 10.4 shows a list of companies that pioneered the development of various antibody technologies for generating chimeric, humanized, and human antibodies and the pharmaceutical companies that acquired them.

Other examples of large pharmaceutical companies acquiring antibody technologies developed by biotech firms include Roche's acquisition of Glycart for $266, which had developed a technology to increase the efficacy of antibodies to kill tumor cells by modifying their carbohydrate moiety (see Chap. 4); GlaxoSmithKline's acquisition of Domantis for $385 million to develop products based on single antibody variable domains; and Amgen's acquisition of Micromet for $1.16 billion, which had developed single-chain bispecific antibodies for harnessing T cells to destroy tumor cells.

10.9   From Antibody Technology Platforms to Product Candidates

Many of the major advances in establishing antibody technology platforms have been made by scientists in academic institutions who founded biotech start-ups to further develop their technology and create novel products. If they are lucky, the

Table 10.4 Acquisition of firms with novel antibody production technologies

Technology	Development firm	Takeover firm
Chimeric mAbs und expression of mAbs	Celltech	UCB
	Genentech	Roche
Humanized mAbs	Applied Molecular Evolution (AME)	Lilly
	Facet Biotech (PDL BioPharma Spin-off)	Abbott
	Idec	Biogen Idec (Fusion)
Human mAb-libraries/ phage-display	Cambridge Antibody Technology (CAT)	AstraZeneca
Human mAbs from transgenic mice	Abgenix	Amgen
	Medarex	Bristol-Myers Squibb

scientists catch the attention of rich individuals or large companies who are able to invest substantial amounts of capital with a long-term commitment. More often, however, without the help of someone like Robert Swanson as business manager (co-founder of Genentech), the scientists are confronted with the whole new world of business plans, financial planning, and venture capital. The technology has to be "sold" to interested venture capitalists (VCs) with attractive and convincing presentations. This first step is often the easiest, since venture capitalists operate by spreading their investments over many companies in the hope that a few of them will succeed and eventually be profitable enough to more than compensate their losses. It is then up to the biotech company to validate its technology by developing therapeutic product candidates and attract further investments in subsequent financial rounds. The gut instinct and imagination of investors often play a crucial role. For example, Ablynx co-founder Serge Muyldermans recounted how investor interest in his technology for generating small domain antibodies from camels was moderate until Ablynx came up with the idea of naming them "nanobodies." Thereafter, the company was overrun by the rush of potential investors.

The goal of most biotech companies with the technology to develop therapeutic antibodies is to acquire sufficient capital to take the most promising product candidate through clinical phases I and II. If the results of these clinical studies are convincing, it stands a good chance of being in-licensed from a large pharmaceutical company with the financial resources to carry out phase III clinical studies (see below). To secure the entire platform technology and avoid competition from other firms, the pharma company often acquires the entire biotech company.

10.10   From Product Candidates to Therapeutics

Clinical Trial Approval

The safety standards for clinical trials of novel antibody products were rigorously revised after the TeGenero catastrophe (see Chap. 6). To better assess the risk of a strong side reaction in humans, toxicology studies are carried out where possible in primates. After the administration of increasing amounts of the therapeutic agent, the side effects are investigated by taking tissue samples and measuring clinical parameters. Such studies are only useful if the antibody also binds to the corresponding animal antigen, which is why most antibody firms try to generate cross-reactive antibodies. If this is not possible, there are two alternative animal models employing either transgenic animals or a surrogate antibody.

In the transgenic animal model, the gene of the human target antigen is integrated into the genome of an animal (usually a mouse or a rat). The success of this procedure depends on the complexity of the target molecule. In the case of bispecific antibodies where two human genes have to be integrated into the genome, this is a difficult and time-consuming undertaking. For the surrogate animal model, an antibody with the same general structure and properties as the therapeutic antibody has to be generated that binds the corresponding antigen of the animal model.

If the developer does not succeed in establishing any of the above animal models, he has a particularly tough stand with the approval authority. A lot of in vitro data is required, and, if a clinical study is approved at all, the phase I study to investigate the safety of the product must start with almost homeopathic amounts of the therapeutic agent, which are gradually increased to therapeutically meaningful levels. This process can take up to 2 years, a time horizon that is usually too long for investors of small biotechnology companies; other projects with the possibility of a faster return are usually preferred. If a relevant animal model is available, the phase I study is usually completed after 1–2 years with the participation of 20–80 patients.

After the phase I study, the proof of concept (POC) to provide evidence of therapeutic efficacy and the optimal dosing strategy is investigated in a phase II study. This phase is often carried out in two separate clinical trials (phases IIa and IIb). The phase IIa clinical trial is a relatively small study to investigate efficacy, potential utility, and common short-term side effects and the effective dosing range. Phase IIb clinical trials are carried out with a larger number of patients with the goal of further evaluating efficacy and safety and to better define the optimal dosing regimen. Phase II clinical trials take about 2–3 years with 50–200 patients. Finally, a large phase III study lasting 3–5 years is carried out to demonstrate significant therapeutic efficacy compared to standard treatment and to investigate the frequency and severity of potential side effects. This trial requires 200–1000 or more patients in several centers and usually costs several hundred million dollars. This trial is often termed a pivotal clinical trial (sometimes termed "registration studies") since it aims to provide sufficient evidence of efficacy for market approval. Interestingly, the FDA appear to have loosened their criteria for the clinical testing of certain product candidates in the last few years, since an increasing number of phase II studies are being accepted as pivotal studies. Extra data are sometimes generated during the reviewing process in a phase IIIb clinical trial which are not necessarily required for market approval but which provide additional drug profile data.

10.11   Help from MABEL to Calculate the Starting Dose

The calculation of an appropriate starting dose is often a contentious point between institutions that approve clinical studies and the applicant. The higher the starting dose, the faster the phase I study can be carried out with lower costs. Prior to the TeGenero disaster, the starting dose was often a tenth of the calculated NOAEL ("No Observed Adverse Effect Level"). After TeGenero, the NOAEL was still an important parameter but not decisive, since the primates used in the study tolerated relatively high amounts of the product without serious side effects. The EMA ("European Medicines Agency") therefore proposed the "Minimal Anticipated Biological Effect Level" (MABEL) for the initial dose. This is a value calculated not only from animal experiments but also from in vitro studies. In the case of antibodies, if the product is highly active at low concentrations and the mode of action of the targeted molecules is not well-known, the drug is classified as a high-risk product, which can only be administered with very low starting doses. The data from the animal models must also be shown to be relevant for humans. Antibodies against two molecules (dual-binding or bispecific antibodies) are almost always classified as high risk. Similar stringent criteria for the calculation of the FIH ("First in Humans") dose are required by the FDA.

10.12 Cost Containment: NICE to Have?

A recent report by Wellcome and IAVI (International Aids Vaccine Initiative) pointed out that about 80% of the global market for mAbs is represented by the United States, Canada, and Europe. A major factor limiting their general accessibility is the high cost. For example, the median price of monoclonal antibodies for 1 year of treatment in the United States in the area of oncology/hematology in 2019 was about $143,000. National governments are increasingly reluctant to accept the prices dictated by the pharma industry. In negotiations with pharmaceutical companies, one of the most common price control mechanisms is to use an international reference pricing (IRP) that compares the proposed prices in several countries. In the case of countries with potentially very large markets such as China, pharmaceutical companies are often prepared to accept significant price reductions.

An approach used by more than 25 European countries is to establish cost-effectiveness thresholds using health technology assessment (HTA) mechanisms to facilitate decisions regarding reimbursement. In Great Britain, for example, cost-benefit calculations for drugs are carried out by the National Institute for Health and Care Excellence (NICE), which was founded in 1999 as an advisory organization by the Ministry of Health and served as a model for other European countries. It uses the costs per quality-adjusted life years (QALY) as a measure of cost-effectiveness that reflects not only the gain in length of life but also the gain in the quality of life.

10.13 QALY

The QALY is measured on a scale from 0 to 1. For example, if the quality of life is doubled (e.g., from 0.3 to 0.6) and the average life expectancy is increased from 1 year to 1.5 years, the QALY is $(1.5 \times 0.6) - (1.0 \times 0.3) = 0.6$. If treatment with the new drug costs €12,000 more than the old drug, the cost of the improved QALY is €12,000/0.6 = €20,000. In this example, the costs are below the limit for an acceptable cost-benefit ratio of around €26,000–€36,000. In the case of Avastin for the treatment of colon cancer, this limit was clearly exceeded. NICE therefore advised the National Health Service (NHS) not to cover the treatment costs. The cost of Kadcyla, Roche's antibody-drug conjugate for the treatment of breast cancer, was also rated as exceeding the threshold by NICE. These calculations can be used to find a compromise with pharmaceutical companies. However, the European Consortium in Healthcare Outcomes and Cost-Benefit Research (ECHOUTCOME) recommended not using the QALY to make healthcare decisions but to focus on the costs per relevant clinical outcome on an individual basis. NICE responded that in its opinion, QALYs are better than any of the proposed alternative measures.

10.14 Cost Reduction with Biosimilars

The patents for many high-revenue biopharmaceutical products have expired or will soon expire. In Europe, for example, MabThera/Rituxan and Herceptin are no longer protected by patents. However, the prices for many antibodies going off-patent are not expected to plummet as is often the case with conventional small chemical drugs since the development and production of biosimilars is still a costly process. Furthermore, therapeutic antibodies are complex molecules whose heterogeneity, binding properties, and mode of action can be significantly influenced by the manufacturing process. Extensive clinical testing is therefore still necessary to ensure that the efficacy and safety profile are comparable to those of the original product. In many countries, biosimilars are generally only 10–35% less expensive than the original product.

Selected Literature

Bourrilly C. Antibody therapeutics: business achievements and business outlook. In: Little M, editor. Recombinant antibodies for immunotherapy. 1st ed. Cambridge: Cambridge University Press; 2009. p. 374–402.

Feng R-M, Zong Y-N, Cao S-M, Xu R-H. Current cancer situation in China: good or bad news from the 2018 global cancer statistics? Cancer Commun. 2019;39:22. https://doi.org/10.1186/s40880-019-0368-6.

Global Cancer Observatory: Cancer Today. Lyon: International Agency for Research on Cancer. https://gco.iarc.fr/today.

Henley SJ, Thomas CC, Lewis DR, et al. Annual report to the nation on the status of cancer, part II: progress toward healthy people 2020 objectives for 4 common cancers. Cancer. 2020;126(10):2250–66. https://doi.org/10.1002/cncr.32801.

Howlader N, Noone AM, Krapcho M, et al., editors. SEER cancer statistics review, 1975-2017, Bethesda, MD: National Cancer Institute, based on November 2019 SEER data submission, posted to the SEER web site, April 2020. https://seer.cancer.gov/csr/1975_2017/.

IAVI/Wellcome. Report: expanding access to monoclonal antibody-based products: a global call to action; 2020.

Kaplon H, Muralidharan M, Schneider Z, Reichert JM. Antibodies to watch in 2020. MAbs. 2020;12(1):1703531. https://doi.org/10.1080/19420862.2019.1703531.

Noone AM, Howlader N, Krapcho M, et al., editors. SEER cancer statistics review, 1975-2015. Bethesda, MD: National Cancer Institute; 2018, based on November 2017 SEER data submission, posted to the SEER web site. https://seer.cancer.gov/csr/1975_2015/.

Origin of biotechnology—a Genentech perspective (from Genenlab notebook, 1996). http://blog.zymergi.com/2013/01/origins-biotech-genentech.html.

Wu S, Powers S, Zhu W, et al. Substantial contribution of extrinsic risk factors to cancer development. Nature. 2019;529:43–7.

Outlook

11

Abstract

The remarkable results achieved with antibodies directed against immune check-points for the treatment of some solid tumors has highlighted the importance of understanding the biology and mechanisms of cellular interactions within the tumor microenvironment (TME). A majority of antibodies in development for treating cancer are directed against immune checkpoints (ICs). They are being evaluated in more than 3000 clinical trials as first or second lines of treatment, alone or in combination with other antibodies and reagents for the treatment of about 50 types of cancer. The percentage of antibody-drug conjugates (ADCs) has also significantly increased within the last decade. Major improvements have been made in linker chemistry and payload efficacy. A large number of bispecific antibodies and chimeric antigen receptor T cells (CAR-Ts) are also now being clinically evaluated, and personalized tumor vaccines could play an increasingly important role. Future cancer therapy involving antibodies will most likely comprise a combination of different approaches devised according to our knowledge of the tumor's immunobiology and its interaction with the tumor microenvironment.

11.1   Introduction

The sales revenue for the Roche blockbusters Rituxan/MabThera (lymphoma and leukemia), Herceptin (breast cancer), and Avastin (solid tumors) were a major incentive for other biotechnological and pharmaceutical companies to produce similar and even more effective products. Human or humanized anti-HER2 antibodies and mAbs to various growth factors are being developed to produce better (or cheaper) alternatives to Herceptin and for treating other solid tumors. Attempts are being made to break the hegemony of Avastin by developing antibodies against other factors and receptors that promote the growth of tumor blood vessels such as VEGFR2 and PDGFRA.

To generate an improved follow-on product for Rituxan, Roche developed the humanized glycoengineered antibody Gazyva (obinutuzumab), which binds the CD20 antigen more effectively than Rituxan to generate a stronger apoptosis signal. It also binds the Fc receptor on NK cells with higher affinity due to its reduced fucose content, thus resulting in an improved ADCC. In in vitro tests and xenograft animal models, it performed significantly better than Rituxan. However, in clinical trials, the in vitro efficacy was not reflected in much better outcomes. In the phase III "Gallium" trial for the treatment of follicular lymphoma, although Gazyva significantly prolonged progression-free survival in combination with chemotherapy for previously untreated patients, the overall survival compared to Rituxan (plus chemotherapy) was similar. Furthermore, in the "Goya" trial for the first-line treatment of previously untreated patients with diffuse large B-cell lymphoma (DLBCL), Gazyva did not extend progression-free survival when combined with the chemotherapy regimen CHOP in comparison to Rituxan/CHOP.

11.2   A New Generation of Antibodies for Cancer Therapy

Many of the antibodies in the new generation of antibodies for cancer therapy are directed against immune checkpoints and used either alone or in combination with other reagents. Outstanding results have been achieved for the immunotherapy of some solid tumors that were previously unresponsive to any kind of treatment. Furthermore, a multitude of novel antibodies carrying cytotoxic payloads, antibodies targeting the tumor microenvironment (TME), and antibodies for harnessing cytotoxic immune cells are providing new angles for attacking the Achilles' heels of diverse cancers. A list of mAbs in late-stage clinical trials that could come onto the market in the next few years is shown in Table 11.1.

11.3   Targets of mAbs in Late-Stage Clinical Development

Many of the targets for the antibodies shown in Table 11.1 are antigens for already approved mAbs or are relatively well-known as potential cancer targets. The predominant targets are clearly immune checkpoints. In addition to the clinically validated targets PD-1, PD-L1, and CTLA-4, antibodies directed against the immune checkpoints LAG-3 and TIM-3 are showing promising results in clinical studies.

LAG-3

LAG-3 (lymphocyte-activation gene 3) is expressed on T effector cells and T regulatory cells (Tregs). Binding to its primary ligand MHC class II results in the suppression of T effector cells and the upregulation of Treg activity, thus creating a

Table 11.1 Monoclonal Abs in late-stage clinical studies for cancer therapy

INN/code name	Molecular format	Target	Phase	Indications
Belantamab mafodotin	Huz IgG1 ADC	BCMA	2 piv.	Multiple myeloma
Oportuzumab monatox	Huz scFv immunotoxin	EpCAM	3	Bladder cancer
Margetuximab	Ch IgG1	HER2	2/3; 3	Gastric/ge; breast
Dostarlimab	Huz IgG4	PD-1	3	Endometrial cancer; ovarian cancer
Spartalizumab	Huz IgG4	PD-1	3	Melanoma
131I-omburtamab	Mu mAb, radiolabel	B7-H3	2/3	Neuroblast/leptomen
Loncastuximab tesirine	Huz IgG1 ADC	CD19	2 piv.	DLBCL
Balstilimab	Hu IgG4	PD-1	2 piv.	Cervical cancer
Zalifrelimab	Hu IgG1	CTLA-4	2 piv.	Cervical cancer
Utomilumab	Hu IgG2	4-1BB	3	DLBCL
SAR408701	mAb ADC	CEACAM5	3	NSCLC
MT-3724	scFv immunotoxin	CD20	2#	DLBCL
REGN1979	Hu IgG4 bisp.	CD20, CD3	2#	Follicular lymphoma
Camidanlumab tesirine	Hu IgG1 ADC	CD25 (IL2RA)	2 piv.	Hodgkin lymphoma
AFM13	Bisp. tandem diabody (TandAb)	CD30, CD16A	2 piv.	Periph. T cell-lymph.
TJ202, MOR202	Hu IgG1	CD38	3	Multiple myeloma
131I apamistamab	Mu IgG1, radiolabel	CD45	3	Ablation bone marrow
Zolbetuximab	Ch IgG1	Claudin-18.2	3	Gastric/ge
Tremelimumab	Hu IgG2	CTLA4	3	NSCLC et al.
Cetuximab-IRDye® 700DX	Ch IgG1—IR700 (phototherapy)	EGFR	3	HNSCC
Bemarituzumab	Huz IgG1	FGFR2b	3	Gastric/ge
Daromun (L19IL2 + L19TNFα)	scFv fusion proteins	Fibronectin domain B	3	Melanoma
Mirvetuximab soravtansine	Huz IgG1 ADC	Folate receptor 1	3	Ovarian cancer et al.
Tebentafusp	Bisp. fusion protein	gp100, CD3	2 piv	Melanoma, uveal
[Vic-] trastuzumab duocarmazine	Huz IgG1 ADC	HER2	3	Breast cancer
BAT8001	Huz IgG1 ADC	HER2	3	Breast cancer
Relatlimab	Hu IgG4	LAG-3	2/3	Melanoma
AK105	Huz IgG1	PD-1	3	NSCLC
Camrelizumab	Huz IgG4	PD-1	3	Gastric/ge et al.
HLX10	Huz mAb	PD-1	3	NSCLC et al.
INCMGA00012, MGA012	Huz IgG4	PD-1	2/3	Gastric/ge; HNSCC
Prolgolimab	Hu IgG1	PD-1	2/3	NSCLC
Tislelizumab	Huz IgG4	PD-1	3	NSCLC
MGD013	Hu IgG4 bisp. DART	PD-1, LAG-3	2/3	Gastric/ge
TQB2450, CBT-502	Huz IgG1	PD-L1	3	HNSCC
CS1001	Huz IgG4	PD-L1	3	NSCLC; gastric/ge
Envafolimab	mAb, single domain	PD-L1	3	Biliary tract carcinoma

(continued)

Table 11.1 (continued)

INN/code name	Molecular format	Target	Phase	Indications
Bintrafusp alfa	Hu IgG1 bisp. Conj.	PD-L1, TGFβ	2/3	Biliary tract cancer
MBG453	Huz IgG4	TIM-3	2 piv	Myelodysplastic syndrome
Tisotumab vedotin	Hu IgG1 ADC	Tissue factor	2 piv	Cervical cancer

Source: Kaplon et al. Antibodies to watch in 2020. MAbs.2020:12(1):1703531. doi:https://doi.org/10.1080/19420862.2019.1703531
INN International nonproprietary name, *piv* pivotal, # potentially pivotal, *Mu* murine, *Ch* chimeric, *Huz* humanized, *Hu* human, *scFv* single-chain antibody, *BCMA* B-cell maturation antigen, *Gastric/ge* gastric/gastroesophageal junction adenocarcinoma, *Neuroblast/leptomen* neuroblastoma central nervous system/leptomeningeal metastases, *DLBCL* diffuse large B-cell lymphoma, *NSCLC* non-small cell lung cancer, *HNSCC* head and neck squamous cell carcinomas, *EpCAM* epithelial cell adhesion molecule, *HER2* human epidermal growth factor receptor 2, *EGFR* epidermal growth factor receptor, *VEGF-A* vascular endothelial growth factor A, *CTLA-4* cytotoxic T-lymphocyte-associated antigen 4, *131I* conjugated with iodine-131, *PD-1* programmed cell death protein 1, *PD-L1* PD ligand 1, *FGFR2b* fibroblast growth factor receptor 2b, *B7 H3* B7 homolog 3, *CEACAM5* CEA cell adhesion molecule 5, *TGFβ* transforming growth factor-ß, *LAG-3* lymphocyte-activation gene 3, *TIM-3* T-cell immunoglobulin and mucin domain-containing protein 3

tolerizing microenvironment for tumor growth. Inhibition of LAG-3 has shown synergy with PD-1 inhibition in mouse models, resulting in more robust T-cell responses. One of the mAbs in Table 11.1 is a bispecific antibody targeting both of these immune checkpoints.

TIM-3

TIM-3 (T-cell immunoglobulin and mucin domain-containing protein 3) is expressed on many immune cells and also has numerous ligands such as galectin 9, phosphatidylserine, HMGB1 (high-mobility group box 1 protein), and CEACAM1 (carcino-embryonic antigen-related cell adhesion molecule 1). It is a typical marker for exhausted T cells, and its upregulation on tumor-infiltrating lymphocytes has been correlated with poor outcomes in many different types of cancer. Preclinical data suggest that it may provide a mechanism of resistance to the blockade of PD-1. Combinations of antibodies to TIM-3 and PD-1 or to TIM-3 and CTLA-4 have demonstrated preclinical efficacy.

Claudin-18.2

The predominant targets of antibodies in late-stage clinical development are clearly immune checkpoints. One of the relative "newcomers" is claudin-18.2. Claudins are important components of the tight cell junctions controlling the flow of molecules between cells. In 2008, Uğur Şahin and colleagues described the identification of isoform 2 of claudin-18 as a highly selective cell lineage marker strictly confined to differentiated epithelial cells of the gastric mucosa. Furthermore, it is expressed in a significant proportion of gastric cancers with frequent ectopic expression in pancreatic, esophageal, ovarian, and lung tumors.

Fibronectin Extra Domain B

A splice variant of the extracellular matrix protein fibronectin contains a so-called extra domain B that is almost exclusively expressed by newly formed blood vessels in tumors. The mAb L19, which specifically targets this domain, has shown therapeutic potential when fused with cytokines such as IL-2 and TNFα. Despite severe side effects such as capillary leak syndrome and hypotension, IL-2 has been shown to mediate the regression of some tumors, and it has been approved for the treatment of metastatic renal cell carcinoma and metastatic melanoma. Coupling it with a tumor-specific antibody is expected to make it significantly safer since it will mainly unfold its activity at the site of the tumor. The same holds true for TNFα, whose pro-inflammatory activities appear to synergize with IL-2 in provoking an immune response against tumor cells. Administration of Daromun (Table 11.1, a combination of an L19 scFv fused to IL-2 and an L19 scFv fused to TNFα) may provide an effective means of overcoming the immunosuppressive activity of the tumor microenvironment.

CEACAM5

CEACAM5 (carcinoembryonic antigen-related cell adhesion molecule) is a member of the carcinoembryonic antigen (CEA) family of glycoproteins involved in cell adhesion. Whereas it is only weakly expressed in healthy tissues, it is highly expressed on approximately 20–30% of lung adenocarcinomas and on the surface of some other cancers including colorectal, gastric, and breast cancers.

Folate Receptor 1

Folates are essential for the synthesis of DNA and the synthesis of methionine from homocysteine. The drug methotrexate is therefore often used in cancer chemotherapy since it interferes with folate metabolism. The folate receptor 1 (aka folate receptor α) is often overexpressed by a number of carcinomas including ovarian, breast, renal, lung, colorectal, and brain.

4-1BB

4-1BB is expressed by a number of immune cells including T cells, dendritic cells, B cells, NK cells, neutrophils, and macrophages. In vitro studies showed that stimulation by agonistic anti-4-1BB antibodies resulted in the activation of both CD4+ and CD8+ T cells as well as the activation of APC (antigen-presenting cells) and NK cells. However, in vivo administration of an agonistic antibody in mouse models leads to the deletion of several cell types including B, NK, and CD4+ T cells while promoting CD8+ T-cell expansion. The reasons for this discrepancy are unknown. However, its costimulatory activity on cytotoxic T cells and its ability to induce high amounts of IFNγ make it an attractive target for cancer therapy.

Tissue Factor

Tissue factor (TF) is found on the surface of many extravascular cells, including vascular smooth muscle cells and adventitial cells, which form an integral part of the blood vessel wall. Following injury, TF becomes exposed and builds a catalytic complex with its ligand coagulation factor VII that initiates the coagulation protease cascade. Tissue factor also plays a significant role in some types of cancer, since it can promote tumor growth, angiogenesis, and metastasis. Based on its high expression on many solid tumors and its rapid internalization, tissue factor was selected as a target for the treatment of cervical cancer with an ADC.

11.4 Trends in Molecular Formats of Approved and Late-Stage mAbs

The various antibody formats used since 1995 for cancer therapy are summarized in Table 11.2. Interestingly, most of the mAbs that have been approved since 2015 or that are in late-stage clinical development are humanized mAbs rather than completely human antibodies. This may partly reflect the fact that, despite impressive technologies for generating high-affinity human antibodies, a plethora of well-characterized murine monoclonal antibodies have been generated against all manner of antigens in the previous decades.

A marked trend of Table 11.2 is the increase of mAbs carrying cytotoxic payloads. The delivery and release of cytotoxic payloads conjugated to antibodies have been steadily optimized by advances in the synthesis of improved linkers and the efficacy of payload cytotoxic action. Five of the eight late-stage ADCs employ payloads designed to disrupt microtubules, and three ADCs have payloads that irreparably damage DNA. An increasing number of solid tumors are being targeted by

Table 11.2 Molecular formats of approved and late-stage mAbs

Approved therapeutic Abs						
	1995–2000	2001–2005	2006–2010	2011–2015	2016–2020	Late-stage 2020[a]
Murine	1	2	1	–	–	2
Chimeric	1	1	–	2	1	3
Humanized	2	2	–	4	7	16
Human	–	–	2	6	5	12
Naked[b]	3	3	2	10 (3.IC)	7 (4.IC)	20 (17.IC; 1.Cos)
Radiolabel	–	2	–	–	–	2
Toxin	–	–	–	–	1	2
ADC	1	–	–	2	6	8
Bispecific	–	–	1	1	–	4 (2.IC)
Photolabel	–	–	–	–	–	1
Cytokine conjugate	–	–	–	–	–	1

[a]Data from Table 11.1
[b]*Naked* full-length monospecific mAb without a payload, *IC* mAbs against immune checkpoints, *ADC* antibody-drug conjugate, *IC* immune checkpoint, *Cos* costimulatory Ab

ADCs, and they may achieve even better efficacy in combination with other agents. It may also be possible to increase the amount of cytotoxic payload using nanoparticles targeted to the tumor site with recombinant antibodies.

By far the most striking feature of Table 11.2 is the number of monospecific naked antibodies directed against immune checkpoints in late-stage clinical development. Seventeen of the 20 antibodies are directed against ICs, and one antibody is directed against a costimulatory receptor. Only two of the antibodies are directed against tumor-associated antigens, namely, CD38 and claudin-18.2. The identification of further surface molecules as potential targets for monospecific naked therapeutic antibodies may be facilitated by analyzing the large amount of data that is accumulating on the expression of cell surface proteins (the surfaceome).

11.5 Immune Checkpoint Inhibitors

Antibodies against PD-1 or PD-L1 have become one of the most widely prescribed therapeutics for treating cancer. ICIs are now used alone or combined with chemotherapy as first or second lines of treatment for about 50 types of cancer. Furthermore, they are being evaluated in more than 3000 clinical trials, representing about 2/3 of all such trials for treating cancer. About 20% of patients with melanoma achieve complete responses after being treated with ICIs. Furthermore, the risk of relapse for these patients is estimated to be less than 10% over a 5-year follow-up after discontinuation of the approximately 6-month treatment. Regarding the long-term adverse effects, approximately 10% of patients treated with anti-PD-1 antibodies develop hypothyroidism and need a continuous hormone replacement therapy.

Not all tumors respond as well as melanoma to treatment with ICIs. The most susceptible tumors appear to be those which have been termed "hot tumors" (see Chap. 6). These are characterized by a significant number of tumor-infiltrating cells (TILs), the expression of immune checkpoints, and a high tumor mutational burden (TMB). In future approaches, it may be possible to block the escape mechanisms described in Chap. 6 by devising cancer therapies based on a better understanding of tumor immunobiology and the interactions between tumor and immune cells in the immunosuppressive tumor microenvironment (TME). Another major goal to aim for is the manipulation of the TME to effect a transition from a cold to a hot tumor.

Most of the ICIs in development are for the inhibition of T-cell immune checkpoints. However, inhibition of immune checkpoints in other immune cells could provide other possibilities for cancer therapy, either alone or in combination with other ICIs. For example, further data on the major immunosuppressive pathways used by tumor cells to evade recognition by NK cells could provide a more efficient approach for exploiting their cytotoxic potential. Combinations of antibodies targeting both the ICs of T and NK cells could enable an immune response against tumor cells mediated by both the innate and adaptive immune system.

11.6   CRISPR-Cas9 Gene Editing

CRISPR-Cas9 gene editing is a powerful technology that can change the DNA of cells with single base pair precision. Multiple genes in T cells can be simultaneously targeted with this technology to improve cancer immunotherapy. For example, to construct a CAR-T cell for adoptive transfer into patients, two genes encoding the endogenous T-cell receptor (TCR) chains, TCRα (TRAC) and TCRβ (TRBC), were deleted to enhance the expression of a transduced synthetic cancer-specific TCR. In addition, a third gene (PDCD1) encoding PD-1 was deleted to remove its inhibitory effect on the antitumor T-cell response. The technology has also been used to investigate the ligand binding of a cancer-specific TCR (see Chaps. 3 and 9). In future applications, CRISPR-Cas9 gene editing can be expected to facilitate many other novel immunotherapeutic approaches.

11.7   CARs Versus Bispecific Antibodies

One of the advantages of CARs over bispecific antibodies is that they can be engineered to secrete factors that combat the immunosuppressive TME. For example, CAR-T cells have been engineered to secrete PD-1, CTLA-4, or PD-L1 antibodies or stimulatory cytokines at the tumor site (see Chap. 9). NK cells are also being investigated as an alternative immune cell for the expression of chimeric antigen receptors. In early-stage clinical trials, CAR-NK cells were shown to be relatively safe with inherent antitumor activity.

Compared to bispecific antibodies, CAR-T cells have so far demonstrated a higher efficacy with a better duration of response. However, as long as allogeneic "off-the-shelf" CARs are not available, the high cost of individual treatment favors the use of bispecific antibodies. Furthermore, it may be possible to increase the efficacy of bispecific antibodies by combining them with other therapeutic agents, particularly those targeting immune checkpoints and the TME. For example, the bispecific antibody AFM13 in Table 11.1, which targets CD30 on Hodgkin and Reed-Sternberg (HRS) cells and CD16A on NK cells, showed enhanced activity when combined with the anti-PD-1 antibody Keytruda in a clinical phase 1b trial for the treatment of relapsed/refractory Hodgkin lymphoma. A complete response (CR) rate of 46% and an objective response rate (ORR) of 88% were achieved, whereas in a separate study using Keytruda as a monotherapy, the CR was 22.4% with an ORR of 69%. In this proof-of-concept study, most of the adverse events were low grade and remained manageable with standard-of-care treatment.

11.8 Inhibitors of Epigenetic Changes

Epigenetic modifications affect gene expression without modifying the primary genome DNA sequence. They include DNA methylation, alteration of histone patterns and chromatin structure, and alteration of the expression of microRNAs. Epigenetic changes play a major role in the aberrant expression of tumor-associated genes responsible for malignant transformation and cancer progression. To combat epigenetic changes within cancer cells that provide an escape mechanism by abrogating immune recognition, ICIs may prove useful in combination with enzyme inhibitors. For example, the cancer/testis antigen NY-ESO-1 is only expressed in germ cells, placenta, and some tumors. Furthermore, its potent immunogenicity makes it an attractive target for immunotherapy. However, it has a heterogeneous expression that is negatively regulated by DNA methylation and positively regulated by histone acetylation. Preclinical models suggest that a combination of ICIs with inhibitors of DNA methyltransferases and histone deacetylases would be a promising immunotherapeutic approach.

11.9 Tumor Vaccines

Last but not least, in the futuristic realm of personalized medicine, the RNA-based neoantigen vaccine strategy described in Chap. 3 could provide another powerful tool for cancer immunotherapy. Initial clinical studies suggest that the efficacy of such vaccines could be increased when used in combination with ICIs. The speed with which nucleic acid-based vaccines against COVID-19 were developed and approved demonstrates the practical feasibility of this approach.

Furthermore, as described above and in previous chapters, the identification of a cancer-specific T-cell clone and its binding to tumor cells via the monomorphic MHC class I-related protein, MR1, has opened up new possibilities for vaccination with a ubiquitous tumor ligand (or family of ligands) and for a novel adoptive immunotherapy with engineered cancer-specific T cells.

11.10 Conclusion

A new era of cancer therapy seems to be opening up based on a more detailed understanding of tumor immunobiology and the interaction of tumors with their microenvironment. Future treatments will most likely comprise combinations of various reagents, including vaccines and CARs, using antibodies both for targeting tumors and inducing an antitumor immune response. In the latter case, immune cells can be recruited for the targeted killing of tumor cells and/or by inhibiting immune checkpoints. The challenge will be to devise the best strategy for choosing the optimal combination of reagents.

Selected Literature

Acharya N, Sabatos-Peyton C, Anderson AC. Tim-3 finds its place in the cancer immunotherapy landscape. J Immunother Cancer. 2020;8(1):e000911. https://doi.org/10.1136/jitc-2020-000911.

Bausch-Fluck D, Goldmann U, Müller S, et al. The in silico human surfaceome. Proc Natl Acad Sci U S A. 2018;115(46):E10988–97. https://doi.org/10.1073/pnas.1808790115.

Chiappinelli KB, Zahnow CA, Ahuja N, Baylin SB. Combining epigenetic and immunotherapy to combat cancer. Cancer Res. 2016;76(7):1683–9. https://doi.org/10.1158/0008-5472.CAN-15-2125.

Crowther MD, Dolton G, Legut M, et al. Genome-wide CRISPR-Cas9 screening reveals ubiquitous T cell cancer targeting via the monomorphic MHC class I-related protein MR1 [published correction appears in Nat Immunol. 2020 Mar 2]. Nat Immunol. 2020;21(2):178–85. https://doi.org/10.1038/s41590-019-0578-8.

Danielli R, Patuzzo R, Di Giacomo AM, et al. Intralesional administration of L19-IL2/L19-TNF in stage III or stage IVM1a melanoma patients: results of a phase II study. Cancer Immunol Immunother. 2015;64(8):999–1009. https://doi.org/10.1007/s00262-015-1704-6.

Finck A, Gill SI, June CH. Cancer immunotherapy comes of age and looks for maturity. Nat Commun. 2020;11(1):3325. https://doi.org/10.1038/s41467-020-17140-5.

García-Muñoz R, Anton-Remirez J, Nájera MJ, et al. GALLIUM trial: the tortoise (rituximab) and the hare (obinutuzumab) race. Future Sci OA. 2019;5(3):FSO375. https://doi.org/10.4155/fsoa-2018-0122. Published 2020 Jul 3.

Jung H, Kim HS, Kim JY, et al. DNA methylation loss promotes immune evasion of tumours with high mutation and copy number load. Nat Commun. 2019;10(1):4278. https://doi.org/10.1038/s41467-019-12159-9. Published 2019 Sep 19.

Kaplon H, Muralidharan M, Schneider Z, Reichert JM. Antibodies to watch in 2020. MAbs. 2020;12(1):1703531. https://doi.org/10.1080/19420862.2019.1703531.

Klar AS, Gopinadh J, Kleber S, et al. Treatment with 5-aza-2′-deoxycytidine induces expression of NY-ESO-1 and facilitates cytotoxic T lymphocyte-mediated tumor cell killing. PLoS One. 2015;10(10):e0139221. https://doi.org/10.1371/journal.pone.0139221.

Leung D, Wurst JM, Liu T, et al. Antibody conjugates—recent advances and future innovations. Antibodies. 2020;9(1):2. https://doi.org/10.3390/antib9010002.

Murciano-Goroff YR, Warner AB, Wolchok JD. The future of cancer immunotherapy: microenvironment-targeting combinations. Cell Res. 2020;30(6):507–19. https://doi.org/10.1038/s41422-020-0337-2.

Perrier A, Didelot A, Laurent-Puig P, Blons H, Garinet S. Epigenetic mechanisms of resistance to immune checkpoint inhibitors. Biomol Ther. 2020;10(7):1061. https://doi.org/10.3390/biom10071061.

Pietersz GA, Wang X, Yap ML, Lim B, Peter K. Therapeutic targeting in nanomedicine: the future lies in recombinant antibodies. Nanomedicine. 2017;12(15):1873–89. https://doi.org/10.2217/nnm-2017-0043.

Robert C, Ribas A, Hamid O, et al. Durable complete response after discontinuation of pembrolizumab in patients with metastatic melanoma. J Clin Oncol. 2018;36(17):1668–74. https://doi.org/10.1200/JCO.2017.75.6270.

Sahin U, Derhovanessian E, Miller M, et al. Personalized RNA mutanome vaccines mobilize poly-specific therapeutic immunity against cancer. Nature. 2017;547(7662):222–6. https://doi.org/10.1038/nature23003.

Scaranti M, Cojocaru E, Banerjee S, et al. Exploiting the folate receptor α in oncology. Nat Rev Clin Oncol. 2020;17:349–59. https://doi.org/10.1038/s41571-020-0339-5.

Stadtmauer EA, Fraietta JA, Davis MM, et al. CRISPR-engineered T cells in patients with refractory cancer. Science. 2020;367(6481):eaba7365. https://doi.org/10.1126/science.aba7365.

Villanueva L, Álvarez-Errico D, Esteller M. The contribution of epigenetics to cancer immunotherapy. Trends Immunol. 2020;41(8):676–91. https://doi.org/10.1016/j.it.2020.06.002.

Vitolo U, Trněný M, Belada D, et al. Obinutuzumab or rituximab plus cyclophosphamide, doxorubicin, vincristine, and prednisone in previously untreated diffuse large B-cell lymphoma. J Clin Oncol. 2017;35(31):3529–37. https://doi.org/10.1200/JCO.2017.73.3402.

Xin Yu J, Hubbard-Lucey VM, Tang J. Immuno-oncology drug development goes global. Nat Rev Drug Discov. 2019;18(12):899–900. https://doi.org/10.1038/d41573-019-00167-9.